T0074154

The
Support Group

The

Support Group

Connection, Hope, and Healing
for Patients and Providers

Shanda H. Blackmon, M.D., M.P.H., F.A.C.S.

Mayo Clinic Press

MAYO CLINIC PRESS
200 First St. SW
Rochester, MN 55905
mcpress.mayoclinic.org

The information in this book is true and complete to the best of our knowledge. This book is intended as an informative guide for those wishing to learn more about health issues. It is not intended to replace, countermand, or conflict with advice given to you by your own physician. The ultimate decision concerning your care should be made between you and your doctor. Information in this book is offered with no guarantees. The author and publisher disclaim all liability in connection with the use of this book. The views expressed are the author's personal views, and do not necessarily reflect the policy or position of Mayo Clinic.

To stay informed about Mayo Clinic Press, please subscribe to our free e-newsletter at mcpress.mayoclinic.org or follow us on social media.

For bulk sales to employers, member groups and health-related companies, contact Mayo Clinic at SpecialSalesMayoBooks@mayo.edu.

Proceeds from the sale of every book benefit important medical research and education at Mayo Clinic.

Cover design: D. Soleil Paz
Cover art: © Paitoon/Shutterstock.com

Library of Congress Cataloging-in-Publication Data is available from the Library of Congress.

ISBN 979-8-88770-047-2 hardcover
ISBN 979-8-88770-048-9 ebook

Printed in the United States of America
First edition: 2024

This book is dedicated to my patients, especially those who have suffered from esophageal cancer, and to those who taught me so much during survivorship, either by participating in the support group or online social media or by calling and keeping in touch. You each have taught me how to be a better surgeon and a better person. I am always here for you. You are my compass. Whenever I am lost, I turn to your struggle, because focusing on that sets me straight.

This book is also dedicated to my village of support, led by my husband of twenty-eight years, Matt C. Blackmon. It is a privilege to raise our family with you. You have carved your world around mine so that I can care for my patients, launch the UDD App, and write this book. I love you for that and so many more reasons.

Contents

Author's Note

I am grateful for the opportunity to tell my story and the stories of those I have had the privilege of interacting with during my long career. This book is based on my recollections and experiences; I have done my best to depict actual events as truthfully as recollection permits, to represent everyone and everything faithfully. Some names have been changed to protect privacy, a few scenes have been compressed. Dialogue is recalled to the best of my ability.

The
Support Group

Introduction

've been called a pioneer in thoracic surgery,[1] but as most
people know, progress and innovation are possible only
with teamwork and volumes of support. Having developed specialized multidisciplinary crews for complex esophageal reconstruction,
I know the value of well-run, connected teams and the importance
of support—for both the provider and the patient. This knowledge is
hard-won. Early in my career, I led the Division of Thoracic Surgery
at Houston Methodist Hospital, developing it from scratch. During
this process, resources were limited and patient needs were great.
It was up to me to tackle obstacles and to figure out how to meet
patient needs in a creative fashion. No one was keeping track of the
hours I worked. Did the leadership really know what I was facing?
Did they even care? Exhausted and with twin babies at home, I
was spread thin. I had to find a better solution to survive.

Not that I was the only one who was stretched and under-
resourced. My team was inundated with existing patients who
needed follow-up for their issues and new patients who needed
to be seen. It didn't seem to matter that everyone on staff was
working at full capacity. The patients needed more than we could

physically give. This wasn't about skill or dedication. It was strictly a numbers game.

And then I noticed patients trading stories in the clinic waiting room, sharing not just valuable advice but also the most invaluable of all commodities, empathy and support. That was the genesis of the support group, a safe place where men and women dealing with cancer and its aftermath could talk openly about what they were going through. People could be positive or negative or anything in between, as long as they were real, as long as they provided support for one another.

Support. It's a combination of empathy and compassion. It's respect for someone else's struggles and the desire to provide help in whatever way you can.

The experience of that group changed my outlook on the fundamental role of support in healthcare. It also forms the backbone of this book. In it, I share stories from a diverse group of patients I have had the privilege of treating over my career, as well as the staff I have had the honor of working with. There is the patient I call the Marlboro Man, a rugged individual who, after years of grueling treatment from various doctors, gave up his fight and gave in to what should have been only a minor bump in the road to his recovery. There is Michael, an Iraq War vet and one of my youngest patients, who survived esophageal cancer with the best possible outcome and went on to have the best possible life. There is Tom, a gifted young surgeon who tragically took his own life, as did my colleague Peter. And then there are the staff—the nurses, PAs, residents, and fellow doctors who provided tremendous support to my patients and me, and who, I hope, received it from me in turn. Their stories are included here because support really is the true foundation of healthcare.

Everyone needs support—the capacity we all have to help others endure what they are confronting, the environment we need to get us through our hardest days. That's especially true for everyone who works in the medical community. Physicians and surgeons can succumb to drug abuse, alcoholism, suicide, and depression as a result of the tidal wave of administrative work, patient complications, long and unregulated hours, and constant pressure from administration to meet impossible demands with limited support. One doctor commits suicide every day in the United States, making this the profession with the highest suicide rate. I include their stories too, because while we are always striving, like the tide, to lift all boats, we owe it to everyone to talk about the system that has let down too many people, sometimes with tragic results.

This book is a realistic look at the role of support for patients and providers. And while it doesn't shy away from the grim reality of treating people with life-threatening diseases—and the toll this takes on healthcare providers at all levels—it also contains a strong current of hope. I want everyone to know that we have more power than we know. That with focus, resolve, and an abundance of support and determination, great outcomes can be achieved.

One

The Marlboro Man

On my first day as a thoracic surgeon at Houston Methodist Hospital, I was sitting at my desk on the sixteenth floor of the Smith Building, looking out at the expansive Texas Medical Center, thinking about my career ahead. Only a few years earlier, I had been in the very same room interviewing for a residency in the Baylor College of Medicine's cardiothoracic (CT) surgery program. I had interviewed for general surgery right out of medical school in 1998, when I was young enough not to be intimidated. But that day in Houston in 2002, interviewing for CT surgery, I knew I was among the giants in our field: Dr. Michael Reardon, Dr. Joseph Coselli, and Dr. Ken Mattox, who were practicing under the watchful eye of Dr. Michael E. Debakey. I knew all about these surgeons and what they had accomplished, so I fully understood what a privilege it was just to be in the room with them.

I was coming from a smaller program in Georgia and didn't have years in the lab doing research. But I had years of strong practical experience. Not only was I already sewing the proximal anastomoses (sewing a vein taken from the leg to the aorta, then connecting it to the heart vessels with a suture finer than a human hair) for cardiac bypass grafts, but I'd actually filed a preliminary patent for an intra-aortic balloon occlusion system. I imagine the fact that I was dabbling in such ventures at so young an age made me attractive to the people who had practically invented aortic surgery. It was a slight edge, but I would take it.

I remember being thrilled to meet those illustrious surgeons. They were the surgeons people wrote about, the brave pioneers who invented aortic surgery. I wanted to be like them, to push the boundaries of what was possible, to make an impact in the field and discover novel solutions for my patients. I wanted to change the world for the better, as they had. Little did I know at that time that I would match into the program, train with those surgeons, then watch two great institutions—Baylor College of Medicine and Methodist Hospital—split apart over finances, resulting in the emptying of the sixteenth floor of Smith Building where I had interviewed. Those offices were now occupied by the new Weill Cornell Medical College-affiliated Department of Surgery of Houston Methodist Hospital.

When I started, my new office contained a few remnants from its former occupant, most notably a glass shadowbox display-ing surgical artifacts, including a Sengstaken-Blakemore tube. This historical device, innovative in its day (it is used to stop a hemor-rhage in the esophagus), was now rarely used. On the wall across from that, I hung my diplomas, certificates of training, and board certification. We all did this, decorating our offices with evidence of hard-won accomplishments, representing what we believed to be the best things about us. I've always thought it a shame, though, that we rarely leave room to acknowledge our failures, to respect our mistakes. I'm not sure how we would do this—what sort of plaque our errors would merit—but surely we could all do with reminders of our fallibility, of the times we tried so very hard and yet failed.

Or maybe not. Because some cases you never forget.

My first complex esophageal reconstruction patient was a rugged cowboy who ran his own ranch and had been a sixteenth-round NFL draft pick for the Pittsburgh Steelers. This tall outdoorsman looked like the sort of tough guy who could take on anything the world might offer. But he was no match for the laryngeal cancer he was diagnosed with in his late forties.

I recall the day I met Doyle much the way people remember where they were when John F. Kennedy was shot or when they heard about 9/11. Somehow I knew the moment would mark a before and after, that this relationship would reverberate well into my career.

The first thing I noticed about my new patient was that the skin on his neck was discolored, a deeper shade of red than the rest of his skin. It also had an unusual, almost wooden texture—it felt like bark when you touched it. All of this was a result of poor blood supply, damage from radiation, and a lifetime of smoking.

Other than that, he didn't look like he belonged in a hospital bed. Tan, muscular, and lean, Doyle was the epitome of a toughened individual. But I had underestimated his height; only when he stood up did I realize just what a towering man he was. Doyle had the personality you would imagine might belong to the Marlboro Man: full of pride, self-reliant. Despite what he had been through, he had a physical presence that exuded confidence and strength. Cover up his chest and the hole at the bottom of his neck, and you were looking at a formidable man of power and great spirit.

Prior to coming to Houston Methodist, Doyle had been treated at numerous hospitals, His larynx (voice box) had been removed and a tiny hole had been created to connect the esophagus (the tube that leads from the mouth to the stomach) and the trachea (another tube, also called the windpipe, this one leading from the mouth to the lungs). Years of smoking had given him cancer, and he had undergone multiple rounds of radiation with chemotherapy, but in the end he'd had to have this surgery. This tiny hole allowed him to speak, but speech required an electrolarynx, and special treatment was needed to prevent the hole from becoming bigger as he used it. Unfortunately, in spite of what I am sure were careful instructions, Doyle refused to use the equipment properly and instead stayed out on the ranch tending to his cattle, neglecting his health. Over time, the hole between his trachea and esophagus grew bigger, and fluid poured into his airway when he swallowed, which resulted in pneumonia. This required him to travel to our hospital for a series of surgeries to attempt to close that hole. My colleagues tried taking muscle flaps from his chest and placing them between the esophagus and trachea to create a barrier. Unfortunately, this failed, multiple times.

After surgery, patients are given follow-up instructions, and usually those instructions include a lot of rules—rules that Doyle broke. He wasn't the first patient to defy doctors' orders, nor would he be the last. But Doyle was lacking what many equally stubborn patients have: someone to help him "get with the program" (I've heard more than one patient ally use that phrase). Doyle had daughters and a son, but he didn't let them help with his care. He was the one charged with looking after them—with everyone, really. Doyle didn't have anyone to make sure he knew how important it was to use the electrolarynx. He didn't have anyone to challenge him when he smoked through the hole at the top of his chest or to pressure him to come back for wound checks. It was hardly surprising that a man who stated multiple times that he made every effort to avoid medical teams wouldn't come back for follow-up. And I guess, in retrospect, it wasn't surprising that he would continue to cowboy his way around the ranch without giving his wounds time to heal.

The larger hole that had developed as a result of all this neglect is formally referred to as a tracheoesophageal fistula. This fistula was formed by the abnormal connection between the esophagus and the airway (connecting the tubes through which you eat and breathe). In a normal, healthy person, the esophagus and trachea are not connected, nor is the windpipe cut in half and exposed at the bottom of the neck. The small hole between these two structures created by the surgeons to allow Doyle to speak grew over time because of the large amount of radiation Doyle had received and, alas, from the smoking. Most surgeons can predict this will happen in a patient who has had a lot of radiation, and that is why they try to talk patients into using the electrolarynx to speak. Doyle would have none of it. He wanted to be out on the range with his cattle without needing to carry around a device.

But Doyle was in a perilous condition. Tragically, because of the radiation he had received during his cancer treatment, his fistula would never heal. (He had received about 70 gray of radiation; a gray is the unit used to measure the absorbed dose. For context, the workers at the site of the 1986 Chernobyl nuclear power plant accident received between 0.8 and 16 gray.) Radiation damage occurs long after the treatment as the blood vessels die and the tissue begins to harden and scar. The characteristic woody appearance of his skin signified he had been given a very high dose of radiation, with the goal of damaging the cancerous cells and the blood supply delivering nutrients to the cancer (the very same blood supply that helps keep normal tissue healthy also feeds the cancerous cells). While cutting off the blood supply and damaging the cancer cells with radiation did what we had hoped—it had successfully eliminated the cancer—it had other consequences as well, what we call collateral damage. Now Doyle was struggling with the aftermath of the treatment.

I didn't give Doyle the cancer or the fistula. I didn't light his cigarettes for him or contribute in any way to the early complications that made subsequent treatment harder. But I do consider him to be my worst surgical mistake.

Doyle had had enough of hospitals and wanted to get back to his life. I talked to him at length about the severity of his situation, telling him how the stent placed by the other team into the esophagus to seal the leak had migrated below the fistula. (It turns out the esophagus does not like to have large foreign bodies in it and will work hard to squeeze things out if they don't belong.) I explained that the pressure from the stent would almost assuredly make things worse over time. I wanted Doyle to consent to another operation, this one to remove the stent and repair the fistula. But it wouldn't be easy. The surgery was complex and the recovery grueling. I wanted him to know this before I proceeded.

I spoke to Doyle about how experimental the stents were and how we didn't know all of the bad things that might result from using them. I also talked to him about possibly trying another stent but this time trying to fix it in place to prevent migration. Even that might have consequences, I told him. But he didn't want to hear any of it.

My patient's chest looked like a war zone of scars and indentations. I knew another open surgery would be difficult for him, and he told me he was not ready. He had endured so much that he asked me to think of something that would give him more time, something that would protect his airway while he considered other options. I couldn't blame Doyle for wanting a temporary fix. Nor was this approach unheard of. Sometimes we'll do this for patients to get them stronger so that they can survive larger surgeries. I knew

Doyle really needed another muscle flap to fix the fistula, but even though surgery was the best way to solve the problem, we needed to buy some time for him to recover before undergoing the next major procedure. I conceded that placing another stent to allow his lungs to heal wasn't a bad idea. After all, the constant flow of food and liquid going into his windpipe and lungs made him a poor candidate for the operation he needed.

Unusual situations can require unprecedented and untested solutions. We all understand that. Yet there's a fine line between trying new things on patients—experimenting, in effect—and finding creative solutions. When patients present with typical situations, the solutions are often simple and easy. However, the more complex the wounds and the situations, the more elaborate the fixes need to be. Thinking creatively—imagining measures beyond current practices—can enable elegant solutions. But such solutions may lack scientific rigor.

There are many situations in which a surgeon will tell a patient that nothing can be done. I didn't want to be that surgeon. I told Doyle I had a remedy for his predicament: I could provide him with another stent, which I would tack into place so that it wouldn't migrate. After that, we would try another muscle flap to close the fistula. Unfortunately, working under pressure and with tremendous time constraints, I hadn't thought through all the possibilities with the stent. I just hadn't considered everything that could go wrong when you're trying to fix something that will exert pressure on the structures around it. Just like the constant dripping of water on a rock will eventually erode the stone, even a temporary stent can exert enough force on the bodily structures around it to erode the walls of blood vessels, which can result in serious bleeding—essentially turning the body into a ticking time bomb.

I sutured the stent into place to prevent migration, a procedure called a pexy. Initially, my pexy worked. Although I had never seen this done before, it's since been adopted as common practice. We still do that procedure today to prevent stents from migrating. Doyle felt so good that he was once again able to eat, and he proclaimed that he felt like himself for the first time in a long while. We instructed him to avoid cold liquids, as they would shrink the stent and open the leakage again. We also asked him to avoid hot liquids, which might melt the wall of the lining attached to the metal scaffolding of the stent. We explained to him that sometimes thin liquids might make their way between the wall of the esophagus and the stent, and so he would need to thicken any liquids he consumed to make sure things went in the right direction. We arranged for a speech pathologist to work with him and look at his swallowing under fluoroscopy (X-ray) to make sure things were going down into the esophagus and not his airway. He began to eat before we could complete the evaluation and necessary coaching. Instead of carefully taking note of these precautions and engaging in subsequent testing to determine the safety and position of the stent, hardheaded, stubborn Doyle left the hospital against medical advice, what the healthcare team calls "AMA," before I could get a look at his CT (computed tomography) scans or any follow-up testing could be performed, and went back to his ranch in Oklahoma and the cattle.

Doyle was like many patients. He disliked being far from home and hated being in the hospital. A man of the land who for years had taken care of his ranch, his cattle, and his family, Doyle wouldn't let anyone take care of him. He wouldn't let anyone help him through his ordeal, and he certainly wouldn't let anyone challenge his expectations or his stubbornness. Sadly, for all he had been through—for all this formidable individual had endured throughout his life—it was this obstinacy that contributed to his downfall.

Because Doyle left so quickly after the new stent was tacked in place, I was not able to review his tests until after he was gone. That's when I saw the problem. Unbeknownst to me, he had a rare abnormality called a right-sided aortic arch. Not only was my patient's aorta (the main artery coming off the heart, which supplies blood to the entire body) on the wrong side of his chest, but it took a sharp turn and ended in a bulge—a ring of vessels, called a Kommerell's diverticulum—that was pressing against the stent with every beat of his heart, causing erosion. Such an anatomic irregularity often goes unnoticed because patients have no symptoms; however, patients with a Kommerell's diverticulum have a 4-19 percent risk of aortic rupture and an 11-53 percent chance of aortic dissection.[1] (Dissection is a leak inside the wall of the vessel. A full rupture is blood leaking out of the vessel wall.) In Doyle's case, erosion was inevitable.

After I saw the CT scan, I knew Doyle was in trouble. My panic set in as I repeatedly tried to reach him and urge him to come back. In the meantime, I met with the radiology team to try to make sense of the anatomy. I had never seen it before, but I had seen pictures in textbooks and knew it was a huge problem for the stent. Although we had not acquired any images that would have shown this before the stent was placed, I went back and tried to see if the neck images he had in his chart might have given us a clue. The way his aorta traveled down his chest on the wrong side of the body, followed by that sharp turn, meant there would be unusually high pressure against one area of the esophagus— exactly the area where I'd placed the stent. I went through the possible complications in my mind and worried about how they might manifest. It seemed inevitable that the stent would erode the surrounding blood vessels.

I went back to review all his operative notes and records. There wasn't a single notation about the Kommerell's diverticulum in his chart. This detail likely wasn't mentioned because Doyle had mostly had neck imaging and the diverticulum wasn't a relevant part of his history—until now. It's probable that no one even knew it existed. But now that we knew the diverticulum existed, we had to remove the stent immediately.

It didn't take me long to find him. And I found him in trouble.

Before I could even get him on the phone, Doyle's stent had eroded through his esophagus, and then the stent bored into his aorta. Right after he got back to the ranch, he had to be rushed to a local hospital with blood pulsing from his mouth. My patient, literally bleeding to death, was treated by an Ear, Nose and Throat surgeon—who is not familiar with this type of surgery—to stabilize Doyle enough to get him back to Texas. In this attempt to stabilize, the surgeon inserted gauze into Doyle's mouth. This only stopped the external evidence of bleeding while the internal bleeding continued. Remember, his airway was disconnected and his breathing took place from the hole at the bottom of his neck. Packing his mouth with gauze was a futile attempt, akin to mopping up the floor while the sink is still overflowing. It might have made the healthcare team feel better, but it did nothing to stop the internal bleeding. All that could be done at this point was to secure an airway by placing a breathing tube into his trachea, then fly him back to me with a cooler full of blood transfusing all along the way. He was barely alive when he arrived back at Houston Methodist.

Desperate times call for desperate measures. And sometimes forward thinking prompts us to reach back. That's what we did with Doyle. We turned to an archaic piece of medical technology, the same Sengstaken-Blakemore tube that was displayed in that shadow box inside my office. The Sengstaken-Blakemore tube has three ports on one end and two balloons on the other. One balloon goes into the patient's stomach and is filled with air using one port. The other sits in the esophagus and is inflated with the second port. The remaining port—the gastric suction port—suctions fluid and air out of the stomach when properly placed through the mouth.

There's a risk to using this device, which has hardly changed since its invention in the 1950s. If placed improperly, it can affect the patient's ability to breathe. Not to mention that sometimes one of the balloons breaks, with disastrous consequences. But the real danger is in overinflating the balloons, which can rupture the esophagus or compress the nearby airway. Would these efforts save Doyle, or would they cause more harm? He had lost so much blood by then that I was willing to take the risk. We removed the equipment from its display case on my office wall, cleaned it up, and dropped it down into Doyle's esophagus, filling its balloon with a contrasting medium so we could see the anatomy clearly on a CT scan. Applying pressure to the inside of the esophagus, we inflated the balloon to stop the bleeding.

It worked.

People who lose that much blood rarely live to tell the tale. Doyle went through twenty-three units of blood that day, a tremendous trauma when you consider that, on average, the adult body contains roughly ten units. Once we located the problem, we deployed a different stent inside the aorta (yes, another stent) to stop the bleeding. From there we took him to the operating room (OR) to patch the hole in the aorta, remove much of the damaged esophagus, and replace all the blood that had been lost. We knew he would have to undergo reconstruction at some later point to rebuild a new esophagus out of either his stomach or intestine, but that was a problem for another day. For now, we needed to do some temporary but major damage control.

We wound up diverting his esophagus—instead of ending up in the stomach, the tube was cut short, and we created an opening at the neck where it emptied into a bag. As a result, Doyle was officially in gastrointestinal (GI) discontinuity, which meant that whatever he swallowed went directly into the bag on his neck rather than into his GI tract. This diversion of the esophagus would allow the aorta to heal. But it also meant that none of the food he ate by mouth contributed to his nutrition. Instead, liquid food had to be pumped into a small tube that passed through his abdomen and into the stomach. Doyle, desperate to eat again, hated his dependence on the feeding tube.

As we waited for Doyle to heal, I brought together the people needed to be involved in reconstructing the long length of missing GI tract, and we all began to work to deliver a miracle. We decided to create a new esophagus from his small bowel. I had spent an extra year on staff at MD Anderson as a clinical instructor (we call this a superfellowship now) in order to learn this procedure. The complication we feared most was an intrathoracic anastomotic leakage—essentially, a breakdown in the connection deep inside the chest. No matter how long you have trained, all surgeons worry about leaks. It's the wolf that haunts our sleep. A tiny elevation in the white blood cell count, air pockets in the chest, a low-grade fever, an elevated heart rate, and low blood pressure are all signs that point to a possible leak. To add to the fear, an intrathoracic anastomotic leakage has a mortality rate anywhere from 14 to 40 percent, dependent upon the procedure.[2] We remain vigilant for any of these signs until the patient is far away from the hospital and is thriving.

Unfortunately, Doyle developed a leak after we reconstructed a new esophagus for him. And it was terrible. The proximal anastomosis (the connection closer to the mouth) completely fell apart. The high dose of radiation he had received was likely the reason for this, but it was up to me to fix the problem, and I didn't know how. It didn't seem to matter what I did, because the radiated tissue would not heal. I should have known that. And because his anatomy was different—due to the Kommerell's diverticulum—a difficult case was made even more difficult. First I tried stenting the esophagus farther away from the blood vessels (yes, we went back to the stents once again). Then, even though he had already undergone several attempts at flaps to try to repair the fistula prior to my meeting him, I tried another.

Finally, we created a new way of delivering blood vessels to the area to help the wounds heal. We connected a loop of the vein in a U-shape, linking one end to the right arm artery (axillary artery) and the other to the right arm vein (axillary vein). In a case such as this, time is the best healer. We waited a couple of weeks for the vein to heal and become stronger. Then we cut the loop in half, which was like diverting a stream to bring water to a dry piece of land. Now this newly routed artery and vein connected with the free piece of skin and muscle, allowing us to create a skin tube covered with muscle as we folded the flap in half. This was how we rebuilt the missing part of his upper esophagus. If it sounds hard, that's because it is.

It was a nearly impossible task and fraught with complications, but Doyle made it through. We all made it through. Though Doyle spent months in the hospital, suffering through several problems with his airway, emergency tracheostomy changes, and a number of touch-up procedures, his GI tract finally healed, and he could eat once again. We all breathed a sigh of relief. It was a bit of a miracle. It had taken training, science, thorough knowledge of surgical principles, and a lot of thought, but it seemed miraculous to see him completely healed and able to eat, considering how awful his situation had been at times.

A year later, however, Doyle came back with a urinary tract infection. But he refused an antibiotic to treat the infection. It was at this point that he asked for palliative care, and he went home to die. In an otherwise healthy patient, a UTI can be an uneventful infection. However, in Doyle's case, refusing treatment was fatal.

I was devastated.

Yes, part of it was the loss of all the work we had done, all the time the team had put in, and how much the team had sacrificed to accomplish all that. And I was sad—even a little angry, perhaps—because it seemed to me that despite all we had done for our patient, he hadn't valued our efforts. Saddest of all was that he didn't see value in continuing his own life anymore. He was not happy with the quality of his life. Just surviving and being technically able to eat was not enough. How else to explain the way that this man, who had tolerated so much, would let something so seemingly minor defeat him?

Doyle's was a tough case, especially coming so early in my surgical career. His case was so complex, even advanced surgeons would have struggled with all the concepts. I think he would have been difficult for any experienced surgeon to manage. Most might have just said no to another surgery and let him die. In time, I was able to push aside my feelings of defeat over my patient's death and started to ask some tough questions.

We had tried so hard to "fix" Doyle, but what had we really accomplished? By all the common surgical benchmarks, he would have been considered a success. The reconstruction of his esophagus and the restoration of his ability to eat, despite what he had endured and how he looked, would be categorized as complete and good. Yet a "successful" surgery does not in itself guarantee a good outcome. The price Doyle paid for spending months in the hospital and undergoing a series of surgeries just to eat again was high. It took a toll on his family. His ranch was neglected. Many of the cattle died. Without him tending to those he cared for, things wilted around him. His world ceased to thrive.

I believed I had been up front with my patient. I had told him what to expect from the surgery—what could go right and, of course, what could go wrong. I had advised him of the possible risks as well as the rewards. But had I taken everything into consideration? And had I asked the right questions? Had I even considered the amount of support he would need or accept? How did we treat him in such a way that when he was finished with all the reconstructions, the only option he saw was to allow himself to die from a treatable urinary tract infection?

I had wanted to repair my patient as best I could. But in the end, the outcome wasn't good enough. I hadn't been able to give Doyle a life that was acceptable to him. I worried that I had taken him down a pathway that he wasn't prepared for, that the patient's bravado and the surgeon's optimism had made for a bad combination. I made myself a promise there and then. Not only would I make sure that all my patients understood the worst-case scenario, but I would ask what mattered most to them. I would remember that surviving a surgery is not the only goal here. It is the quality of life and the satisfaction with the outcome that counts. I needed to paint a better picture of what each patient might look like after surgery to allow them to share in the decision to operate or not.

What does my patient want?

Because in the end, that's the only thing that matters.

Two

The Fledgling

As surgeons, we have a saying: "With bad judgment comes experience, with experience comes wisdom, and with wisdom comes good judgment." I spent a lot of time ruminating over Doyle's case, trying to decipher the costly lessons. Losing him was devastating. Just when we got over one hurdle, another, more challenging one appeared. It didn't matter how creative or diligent we were, because in the end, despite our best efforts, the biggest hurdle we faced was Doyle himself. I didn't know it then, but you can't save a patient who refuses to accept the changes in his life; who won't contribute to his own recovery and rejects the support offered to him. Sometimes people just give up and there's nothing you can do.

I figured things out along the way. But when you're young and just starting out, your mistakes have magnified consequences. It didn't help that I had little support myself. At the time, I was the only person performing thoracic surgery at Houston Methodist Hospital and I was stretched thin. I was essentially a young surgeon on my own, the only one in my specialty at my hospital for the first four years of my practice. I had general surgery residents, the occasional thoracic surgery resident, and a limited team to support me. That was it. Minimally invasive procedures were relatively novel in thoracic surgery, and working through the mouth to the inside of the airway and esophagus was even more innovative. Doing things for the first time, as was frequently the case for us, we rarely had an opportunity to put a routine in place.

Exhausted and with twins at home, I was often lost. No one seemed to be keeping track of the hours I was working or whether I was able to take a break. I was building a division from the ground up and had to develop an entire program from scratch. I had no partners yet and only a small permanent team. There was my physician assistant, Andrea (whom my husband called "Binky" because I depended on her so much). My secretary, Elaine, managed my life as well as my practice and did it all with grace and skill. Libra was my medical assistant in the clinic and served as the glue that held everyone together. Becky, my nurse in the OR at the time, was another valuable ally. She always seemed to be on the lookout for something she thought I might need for the case, such as a refinement she had read about or a piece of equipment she had heard of. And then there was Melana, the representative from Medtronic, the company that made much of the novel equipment necessary for us to pioneer these cases. She spent quite a bit of time in my operating room as well. Determined to help me succeed, she was always there with new technology, offering to train the nurses and watching the operations. We learned together.

Thank God for these women. Without them, I never would have succeeded.

I was on call 24/7, 365 days a year. At least that's what it felt like. Occasionally one of my partners in general surgery would try to cover for me. But when I took time off or went away on a rare vacation, I felt like my patients paid the price. My general surgery partners did their best to cover me, but it wasn't the same as having thoracic surgery partners. Guilt crept in and made me reluctant to take the time I needed. In spite of that, I did try to be completely present when I was at home with my family. That was when I would try to have more quality time with the kids. Time I longed for.

I felt my life crumbling around me. The pressure to succeed was tremendous. I would wake up at 4:30 a.m. just to go in and get my patients' schedules organized. I would review my cases that day—their films, the case steps, the equipment I needed—and prepare to get the team ready. There were always morning conferences and meetings, and during these meetings, the patients would be brought into the operating room. They'd be anesthetized and have their lines and tubes placed so that when I got out of my morning conference I was able to proceed directly into the OR and start operating.

We always prepared the team for what we might require regarding equipment, medications, positioning, and approach. This is called the surgical briefing. Once the patient is prepped on the operating table, we pause and review our checklist. We start each case with a time-out, making sure we have the correct patient, correct side of the body, correct equipment, and correct sequence. We check the patient's medication and allergy list. And we make sure we've given the patient an antibiotic to prevent infection and heparin to prevent blood clots. Forgetting only one detail could have massive consequences. Having the checklist helps, but the responsibility to make sure everything is in order is always mine.

Meanwhile, my husband would wake the children, feed them breakfast, get them dressed, and take them to school. Matt has always been the primary caregiver on weekday mornings; I would try my best to be there for them, fully present, when I got home. At the end of a long day in either the clinic or the OR, I would lend a hand with dinner and do my best to help with things like costumes, school projects, holidays, and making Christmas cards. I also always tried to read to my children every day, cuddling with them every night before bedtime and often falling asleep at the same time they would when exhaustion overtook me. Sometimes I fell asleep even before they did, with the book in my lap. I stopped sleeping well at night, waking at 1:00 a.m. in a panic about all the work that still had to be done. That's when I started the terrible habit of going to bed early and waking in the middle of the night to try to get caught up.

I needed support but didn't know where to turn.

The chief of our department was a brilliant woman at the top of her field. I loved the idea of having her as a mentor, but the reality was very different. Hands-off in her leadership style, she was, in her own words, a "hippie parent." What that meant was that she gave us a lot of freedom, a lot of room to figure things out on our own. She would say things like "grow where you are planted" and "follow your bliss," but wouldn't share granular or logistic advice. When it came to strategies for getting a grant, succeeding in practice, problem-solving, or navigating critical areas that would define our careers, we were on our own. Had I been a midcareer surgeon, I would have appreciated the opportunity to build my program organically. But I was just starting out and needed some form of guidance, someone to help me find my way in academic medicine. That was hard to do when my chief of surgery was commuting to Houston from Baltimore. Our one-on-one meetings were limited to two or three times in any given year. It wasn't enough.

I was struggling. I needed a solid group of senior colleagues, people above me in leadership to point out potential errors and give general counsel. I longed for guidance. I wanted to establish a strong foundation on which to build my practice, with a pathway that paved a direct road to success. Many of my surgical partners felt as I did. Because the entire department of surgery was, in effect, a start-up, they too were young and inexperienced. They wanted independence and the ability to navigate their own paths, but they also realized the value of mentorship and support. That was hard to come by when most of the faculty were hired early in their careers, meaning that our department was being built from the ground up, without the gray-haired staff that typically dominate the halls of more established practices and academic departments.

There was no one to advise us on joining cooperative groups for research, building multidisciplinary teams, securing OR time, navigating political issues, getting grants funded, starting clinical trials, or answering important questions for patients. There was no road map. It was up to us to develop it.

Misery loves company, or so the saying goes. I don't know that I believe that, but I recall the relief I felt when I found out that others had similar issues. Sometimes we found comradeship sitting in our offices late at night complaining about the lack of guidance. This would, at times, make me feel better, while at other times it would make me feel more frustrated. I often thought about quitting. I wondered if I had chosen the wrong specialty or the wrong hospital or even the wrong profession altogether. I just didn't understand how other people did it. On the outside, I was considered a tremendous success by others. And, irony of ironies, I was somebody whom others felt they could lean on. I was asked to give talks to inspire other women to go into the specialty. I was held up as an example of what is good.

I felt like an imposter.

I was seen as successful because I kept delivering. A busy surgeon who managed to do research and innovate at night and on the weekends, I was burning the candle at both ends. It wasn't sustainable. I loved my team and was engaged heavily with my patients, but much of my work was pointless and could have been allocated or delegated to others. I needed to learn to be more efficient or I was going to burn out. Luckily, Mike Reardon provided me with mentorship, sponsorship, and allyship. One of the surgeons I had first interviewed with in the Smith Building, he helped me with procedural concerns and technical questions; he even taught me how to do an auto-transplant of the heart for a complex left atrial tumor. (This surgery was later highlighted as the "Humpty Dumpty" surgery on *Grey's Anatomy*. When my children heard that, it was the first time they thought what I did was "so cool.")

But it's not just about skills or hard work. Everyone has their own definition of success. For me it was about providing first-class patient care, about aligning my ideals and values with that of my institution. Dr. Reardon respected that. And because he was a man of integrity—I knew him to be honest and true to himself—I listened closely when he shared his experience and his wisdom. "Keep your circle small," he advised me. "Know that sometimes when you're doing the right thing, you'll be met with more resistance." Perhaps the best advice was the hardest to hear. "The hospitals you work in won't necessarily love you back," he told me, and then continued, "Be careful who you trust—many have a different agenda than yours." How true.

The rocky first years of my practice—when I learned to be on my own, manage complex pathology, deal with complications, and learn from patients—were tough but necessary. As a fledgling surgeon without any senior partners inside my own hospital to guide me in my specialty, I had to learn quickly. I had to learn new skills, plus take what I had been taught in the years before and apply it to new patients and new circumstances. This is called the "white wall" phenomenon, when you get out of training and look around for someone to help but suddenly see nothing but the white walls around you. It's a defining time when you learn to think your own way out of problems and bail yourself out. Basically, it's when you put on your big-girl panties and get to work.

I wanted to master my new craft of minimally invasive thoracic surgery. I also wanted to go further, to become as good at minimally invasive surgery in the chest as I had been in the abdomen. Video-assisted thoracoscopic lobectomy (camera inserted in the chest with small incisions to surgically remove one of the lobes of the lung) was a new concept at the time. Some believed it impossible, such as my professor who thought the whole idea was absolutely ridiculous when we discussed it in my thoracic surgery residency. I didn't go quite so far as to call it "ridiculous," but I did share his worries. Where would be the best places to put the small incisions? How would we get the tissue out through the little openings? And because this surgery is often used to remove a lung that is filled with cancer, could we do it this way without any of the cancerous cells spreading into the nearby tissue as we worked?

We could barely conceive of the idea. That is, until we heard about a few pioneering surgeons who had actually mastered this feat. Dr. Rob McKenna at Cedars-Sinai in Los Angeles and Dr. Scott Swanson at the Brigham (Brigham and Women's Hospital, a major teaching hospital in Boston that is affiliated with Harvard Medical School) were on opposite sides of the country from each other, but they had taken similar paths to determine how to perform minimally invasive lung surgery, including lobectomy. Not only had they figured out how to do it, but they'd mastered the skill and made it look easy.

I flew first to the West Coast to learn under Dr. McKenna, and then to the East Coast to hear Dr. Swanson talk about what he thought he had done wrong, how he could have done it better, and discuss unedited video footage that showed him struggling while performing the surgery. His transparency impressed me. It was because of these two surgeons that I was able to come back to my own home institution and begin to master the craft myself.

I also connected with one of the senior partners in my practice who worked mostly in the abdomen, Dr. Brian Dunkin. He was the one who helped me start doing minimally invasive esophagectomy (removal of the esophagus). Learning how to work on the esophagus without needing to make a huge incision helped me develop the skills I would later need to do the same with other structures within the chest. I learned bit by bit. Having him work with me in the operating room, almost as if I was doing another fellowship in minimally invasive surgery, made me feel safe, protected, and supported in my quest to become an early adopter.

When I started at Houston Methodist Hospital in 2006, initially I felt that I had to try to be good at everything. Since I was building my program from scratch, I had to handle any patient with a thoracic problem who was sent to me. I had to take that call every night, every day, throughout the year. The lack of coverage by any other surgeons, the lack of partners to share my practice with, and the intensity of the practice were taking a toll on me. But there was no turning back.

I had to learn new techniques myself, as well as figure out how to lead others to become comfortable with the new technology we were bringing in. Any mistakes I made had to be my own; it was up to me to figure out how to fix them. I had to defend myself and the thousands of decisions I made daily. I had to own my mistakes and give gratitude and credit to my teams when things went well. I needed to stay safe and open for feedback.

I was developing a team, but it wasn't a dedicated team—it was more like a roster of professionals who rotated in and out of the OR. Some people were intrigued by cardiothoracic surgery and asked to work with me on a regular basis. That was a good start, but other than that, there was very little consistency, and so no routine. It seemed like every day there would be a new person in the room, a new person who needed to become familiar with our pioneering process. Variety may be the spice of life, but not in the OR.

The nurses I worked with in Houston identified as cardiac nurses, which meant that additional training was necessary. They were keen and dedicated, and I wanted them to feel that they were part of something, so I bought scrub tops for them and had their names monogrammed on them, and, of course, the name of the unit, "Thoracic Surgery." And because I believed it was vital for us to get to know each other outside the pressurized environment of the OR, I invited them all over to my house, where my husband and I cooked dinner—steak on the backyard grill.

At some point in the days prior to that get-together, I had given everyone a copy of a *Harvard Business Review* article called "Speeding Up Team Learning."[1] The article, which studied cardiac surgical teams at sixteen major medical centers, listed "a team's ability to adapt to a new way of working" as a key determinant of performance. I liked that message, which I felt would be empowering to these professionals who were taking their skills to a whole new level.

I wanted my fledgling team to read the research for themselves, to see how the researchers determined that success in learning new minimally invasive techniques was about more than the expertise of the surgeon leading the group. It was about "the way teams were put together and how they drew on their experiences—in other words, on the teams' design and management." A good team was about more than the sum of its parts. A good team fostered a respectful environment of psychological safety, strong communication, and innovation. It was important for them to know that.

How great, then, to see a number of the nurses sitting around discussing the article that night at dinner. A few had even brought printouts with them, with passages highlighted and underlined. There was a lot of excitement about what we were going to learn, and I was particularly pleased to see how we were bonding. It wasn't just the nurses. My new younger partner, a few residents, my physician assistant, and my secretary came, as did the nurse manager and the scrub tech. I was thrilled to see one of the more senior nurses, Sosama, enjoying herself. She had intimidated the heck out of me when I was a young resident. Tying up the back of my surgical gown, she would announce, "I am the boss of you." That's something you never forget. Sosama had supported one of the most demanding cardiac surgeons before working in my room, and I think some of that culture had come with her. It took a long time to soften her up, but this dedicated nurse, very good at her job, also turned out to be a tremendous ally.

A number of my colleagues were surprised when I told them about the evening, but I wanted to cook good food for my team because that's what you do for people you care about. I valued these people, just as I valued my patients. I needed them to be on board for me to succeed—success, of course, being a healthier patient—and for our patients to thrive. I also wanted them to enjoy working with me because I knew that would mean that they felt valued. I was willing to do almost anything to build a good team. I wanted to do it with support and allyship, not fear and intimidation. I wanted this to be collaborative.

This pioneering new field I was entering did more than implement new procedures and equipment. It was upending the order of the operating room, shifting it from a top-down model to a more collaborative system. The nurses seemed to know this intuitively; one even quoted the article. "Look," she said, "it says here that 'new technology requires greater interdependence and communication among team members.' Amen to that."

I got a little chill when she said that. And I was thrilled to see that one person had highlighted a favorite passage of mine: "Much of the information about the patient's heart that the surgeon traditionally gleaned through sight and touch is now delivered via digital readouts and ultrasound images displayed on monitors out of his or her field of vision. Thus, the surgeon must rely on team members for essential information, disrupting not only the team's routine but also the surgeon's role as order giver in the operating room's tightly structured hierarchy."

Without exception, everyone in the unit had to be made aware of their role as a skilled individual *and* a member of the team—especially a member of the team. I wanted to create a collaborative environment and a level playing field in which people knew they could speak up if they saw something was amiss. My team has saved me more than once, such as the time I left a sponge inside a patient's chest. (Yes, that really happens.) I had just stepped out of the OR to let the plastic surgery team close the chest when a nurse chased me down the hallway to bring me back so that I could remove the sponge before the resident closed up. We're all imperfect. We all need help. So why not encourage an atmosphere of candor and honesty, where people can say what they need to say without fear of repercussions?

That means having team members know you won't get angry and throw a spleen across the room if they correct you. (That actually happened. A beloved but volatile surgeon became so enraged at team feedback that he threw the organ across the OR.) This means our nurses feel free to speak up when they see something wrong. They feel empowered to tell you something and do not feel like they will be punished for making a statement. They feel like their thoughts and opinions are recognized as valuable input for the team. The same goes for anesthesia staff and others who might come into the room.

I felt proud of the team I was building. I wanted people to feel respected and to know that with autonomy comes accountability, which meant that everyone had to be aware of their roles and responsibilities.

Nobody would be micromanaged in my new team.

And everybody would be supported.

Three

The Other Side of Fear

My husband and I had always wanted children. What better way to share our love and build our family? Life can be hard, and I was a little scared about bringing children into an unforgiving world where there is so much to fear. But there's also so much to celebrate—beauty and joy, generosity and kindness. Love. We're both hopeful people at heart, so in the end there wasn't really much of a debate. Still, having children is a special conundrum for the female cardiothoracic surgeon, and we delayed childbirth in the early years of our marriage, thinking there would be a time when we'd have more control over our lives, meaning a better time to have children. Who were we kidding? There's never a perfect moment to start a family. The children arrive and you deal with the chaos with love and good intentions.

I was in the middle of my general surgery residency when Matt and I decided to try for children. I tried not to let the added responsibility scare me. I didn't want fear to get in the way of my dreams. Unfortunately, something else got in the way: I found myself unable to conceive. That meant in vitro fertilization treatments were in order. Very expensive treatments. After doing my research, including talking to friends and acquaintances who had undergone the process, I figured that I might have to undergo five rounds. At $10,000 each, that meant approximately $50,000 at a minimum. This was extra money we needed on top of our living expenses.

Since my husband and I didn't have tens of thousands of dollars tucked under the mattress, we needed to think creatively. At one point we looked at my monthly salary and discovered that, no matter how we tried to fit it in our budget, we simply couldn't afford it. That meant signing up for extra jobs, even though my work hours were already on the wrong side of extreme. One of these assignments was procuring kidneys for organ transplantation for a company called LifeLink. Another was collecting patient histories and conducting physical exams on children in the pediatric emergency room at Children's Scottish Rite Hospital. That was a lucrative job, so if I did a stint at Scottish Rite, I could earn more in a weekend than I could in an entire month of my residency.

Then there was the job I took as the NASCAR pit doctor.

I'd already had some experience with NASCAR. During my intern year of residency, I, along with others in my group, had been assigned to the hospital's trauma bay. Our hospital covered the races and received trauma patients from the racetrack. In addition to the big races, the Atlanta Motor Speedway allowed rookie drivers to drive in an ARCA race—it was sort of like the minors in baseball. In August 1998, a multicar crash occurred during the first lap of one of those ARCA races, the Georgia Power 200 stock-car race. Thirty-year-old Chad Coleman hit a wall almost head-on.

It took track safety officials nearly thirty minutes to cut the driver out of his flaming car. Emergency services placed a collar around his neck, stabilizing his cervical spine and immobilizing him. My co-residents Jeff Schwab and Ralph Breslaw were at the track—Jeff was there on a date with his fiancée, Katie, and Ralph was working as pit doctor that day. When Ralph heard on the radio what had happened, he knew he was going to need all the help he could get, and he called to Jeff, who was nearby, for help. After the EMS team transported Chad from the track to the pit hospital, Jeff and Ralph did their best to care for him, placing bilateral tubes in his chest and examining him from head to toe. Chad was getting the best possible medical attention. Unfortunately, he had sustained a catastrophic head and neck injury.

Despite the use of central lines, fluid resuscitation, and chest tubes, as well as nonstop CPR (cardiopulmonary resuscitation), medical staff worried that Chad wasn't going to make it. He was unresponsive and had suffered extreme trauma. Yet NASCAR officials and the medical crew elected to have him airlifted to the trauma center at Georgia Baptist in Atlanta, where he could have every chance for a resuscitation—and, if it became necessary to pronounce him dead, it would be done with his family there, far away from the racetrack with its ESPN crews and crowds. This seemed so much kinder to his loved ones, and also to the spectators at the Atlanta Motor Speedway.

Chad arrived in our trauma bay with blood everywhere. He was accompanied by Jeff Schwab, who had flown with him on the helicopter doing CPR and whose dress shirt and jeans were now covered in blood. The chest tubes did not have much blood coming from them anymore, but it was clear that something was wrong with Chad's neck or head, as he was bleeding from the ear. I stood at my patient's head and looked down at his face, seeing his features upside down. He didn't respond, move, or blink. Then I examined his eyes and found that his pupils were dilated—they wouldn't constrict even when exposed to bright light. In spite of that, we followed protocol and did everything we could. Amid ongoing CPR, I gently stabilized the head and temporarily removed the cervical spine collar, keeping the head exactly where it had been, so that I could feel the back of his neck for a step-off. The step-off indicates the spine is out of alignment and might be disconnected, broken, or in the wrong place. If this is missed and it affects the spinal cord, a patient can end up with paralysis. Almost every time we did this, there was no step-off—but today there was. I palpated the step-off and felt the head move in an unnatural way. Clearly it wasn't attached to anything stable; the entire spine had been torn in half, and the only thing that was left was the skin holding his head onto his body. I thought about how it might have happened, and realized that during the accident his body had been restrained by the seatbelt, but the head was not. We would later meet with the NASCAR teams about this exact detail. In the next three years, Dr. Robert Hubbard would invent the HANS device, a head restraint that minimized the risk of whip-like head and neck movement in the event of a crash. Tragically, that would come too late for Chad Coleman.

In the trauma bay, we started transfusing blood with a rapid transfuser, alternating bags of blood with bags of crystalloid fluid, for hydration. Almost every trauma patient automatically gets around two liters of crystalloid fluid upon arrival, which helps maintain blood pressure when there has been loss of blood. The clear fluid poured into Chad's central vein—and immediately poured out of his ear. At first I thought it was cerebrospinal fluid, which is also clear. But when we switched the rapid transfuser to blood, it efficiently pushed the blood into his body. With good CPR being performed by the trauma team, infused blood and fluid continued to circulate and that too immediately came out through the left ear. I watched the cycle happen several times until it was very clear: everything that went into his central vein was coming out of his ear. His eyes were a pale blue-green and his pupils were large and black. I will never forget them.

Pronouncing someone dead is never easy. I remembered thinking that this man looked somewhat like my husband, but with blond hair. It was such a strange detail to notice, and even stranger to remember all these years later. I wasn't trying to personalize this death. I knew better than that. But there was something about the way my patient was struck down in his prime, doing what he loved, that haunted me. I couldn't understand the appeal of NASCAR or of any of what I considered to be daredevil sports. Nor could I understand those lone wolves, as I thought of them—people who like to go it alone, to challenge themselves to go faster than the guy next to them. Then, all of a sudden, I realized this wasn't much different from surgery. A driver was nothing without their team, and neither was a surgeon.

And even lone wolves have loved ones. Chad Coleman's family and fiancée were in a hospital family room, waiting for a miracle, I guess. I realized that we would have to have a conversation with them about what had happened to him. We told them that we thought he had had a quick death, which was true, but there was no mention of the broken neck, the blood loss, or the clear fluid draining from his ear—I believe that too much detail can be a terrible thing. I hoped that the fact that we continued to perform CPR for almost an hour beyond the time his brain had died would provide them some comfort, but they were so devastated that there was no comfort to be had.

I tried not to dwell on what happened in the car crash, but it was hard not to replay the event over and over. I thought of this young man, how his family would be forever changed. How the NASCAR community must have been affected too. This was when I decided that I wasn't a fan of the sport.

So why, years later, did I take a job as a pit doctor?

Money certainly had something to do with it. Working the track at NASCAR meant I could put aside money for in vitro treatments. After all, I was determined to have a family. I guess you could say I was racing against my own biological clock. There might have been more at play too. This might have been a way for me to face head-on the great discomfort I felt whenever I thought back to what had happened that August day in 1998. After all, I still was having nightmares about Chad's death, which I now recognize to be a form of what's called "second victim" syndrome[1]—in which physicians exposed to terrible traumatic deaths struggle long after the event. Finding the balance between mourning the death of a patient and carrying on is important. I had always promised myself that I would quit the day I lost a patient and did not cry. Feeling the death and thinking about it are always preferred to being numb to it, which is a sign of burnout.

Ironically, the fact that I was not a NASCAR fan was what got me the job in the pit. The hiring director, Dr. Waterman, told me that I was selected as much for my ignorance as my skill. Ignorance, that is, regarding the drivers and their fame. I didn't know who the big names were, nor did I know anything about them. That was a big check in the plus column, apparently, as management was always on the lookout for people who could be objective, who could think clearly when a driver came in injured. I couldn't imagine that any physician would let a famous name get in the way of a clear-eyed evaluation, but apparently this was a concern for my new employers.

After working my first few races, I realized what a unique position I was in. Before the races started, we were flown onto the racetrack by the trauma helicopter. That meant I got to fly directly across Hartsfield Airport, perpendicular to where the planes land;

it was all I could do not to scream as we went right over the airplanes. We then traveled south along I-85, flying directly above the miles of traffic, much of which was headed toward the track. The crowds must have started arriving early in the morning, because by the time I got there the stands were already filling with people (and beer). With my pit doctor pass, I could go anywhere I wanted, so one Sunday morning I started exploring, curious to learn more about these people and their culture. In the center of the track, there was the pit hospital, garages filled with cars and people working on them, the press, a restaurant, a conference room, fire trucks, and hot cement. The sheer noise of the cars on the track was overwhelming. Mostly everyone in the pit area was wearing earplugs.

I walked into the large conference room to find an assortment of men and women of all ages. It wasn't until I remembered it was Sunday morning that I understood that I had walked into a makeshift church. Drivers and their families and friends had gathered, and many of them were singing. They said a prayer, a preacher spoke, and then finally they talked about the race. A blessing was given, and I saw many people holding hands.

I looked at this cohesive, faithful, and supportive group of people and felt humbled. These were not the tough guys portrayed on TV waving bottles of champagne and standing next to women in cut-off shorts. Each driver seemed to be generally concerned about whether or not they would come out of that race alive. They knew what they were up against on the track. They weren't reckless, nor did they set aside their fear. They used it to keep their wits about them and to fuel their desire to win the race and make it safely to the other side.

There's always something on the other side of fear. I was learning that from my patients, some of whom were facing impossible odds with tremendous courage. Sure, they were frightened, but they moved forward anyway, with the help of those they loved. I saw the same forces at work that morning at the racetrack as families appeared to cling to the drivers in the final moments before the drivers went to the pit to get ready to race. I also saw that there was a very tight bond among those racing—the drivers genuinely cared for one another. They were held up by their teams. I was impressed.

Then I walked through the garage and back to the hospital, where a long line of staff and drivers was waiting for me to clean out their ears. The combination of high volume and earplugs meant that impacted earwax was common. So this was to be my calling—cleaning out the ears of the crew and drivers, with meticulous attention to detail.

Once everyone had clean ears, the race began. It was exciting to see the drivers getting into their cars, to feel the energy as the cars zoomed by on the pavement. Eventually, though, there was another accident, and a driver was brought in with a possible head injury. When he came through the door, it was immediately clear to me that some staff treated him slightly differently than they treated other drivers. I thought maybe this was because he was more famous, or a better driver; I couldn't tell exactly, because I didn't know one driver from the others. They all looked the same to me. He sat in the bed in front of me and I began to examine him.

As is usual in the case of trauma, we have to assess whether or not a patient knows who they are, where they are, and what day it is. As part of this mini mental status exam, we may also ask the patient to repeat the phrase "no ifs, ands, or buts" and ask them to name two simple objects, such as a wristwatch or a pencil. But those first three questions go a long way toward allowing us to assess a person's ability to think clearly, and correct answers are considered evidence enough that there is no immediate head injury. Of course, in a pit hospital, time is of the essence. We have to balance the driver's desire to get back out and finish the race and our need to make sure we're not inappropriately releasing an injured driver who may go back out on the track and, because of his own injury, cause further injury to others. It was important to get this right. This wasn't about pronouncing one man fit to drive on his own; this was about letting a driver get back onto the track and join a lot of speeding cars. The wrong decision could potentially place everyone at risk. I took my job seriously. I had seen what could happen.

"Do you know who you are?" I asked. This first question should be the easiest, but not in this case. My patient looked up at me with disbelief bordering on disdain.

"You're joking, right?" he asked incredulously. "Don't *you* know who I am?"

"It's not important that I know who you are," I responded calmly. "It's important that *you* know."

"Come on," he said. "You're not serious." The question had become a sticking point—a point of pride for this driver.

"You bet I'm serious," I said. "And we can do this all day if you like. But I'm not the one who wants to get back to the track."

And with that he gave in and told me his name. (He was very famous.)

I'm glad I went back to NASCAR after Chad Coleman's death. I'm glad I was able to face my discomfort and reevaluate the NASCAR community. I had made assumptions about these people, and I was wrong. The support they provided for one another on that Sunday in the conference-room church showed me another side of them. They weren't lone wolves, stars, or winners, just scared humans getting out there trying to do something unique, living their lives and facing their fears. Just like I was.

Four

The Support Group

I t's a privilege to be part of an efficient, experienced and aligned team. I'm at my best when I partner with collaborative professionals who come together with the best interests of the patient in mind, who live up to their responsibilities, communicate clearly, and respect each other enough to have mature disagreements. That's the type of supportive environment in which everybody thrives—providers and patients alike. Yet there have been times (too many times, alas) when I felt overwhelmed and undermined, when I felt that I didn't know how to solve a problem or even understand what the problem was. I wasn't alone.

My team had more work than we could handle, and we were inundated with existing patients who needed follow-up for their issues. If we gave everyone all the follow-up appointments they requested, we wouldn't have had any room for new cases and the practice would have failed. Which meant that we would have failed everyone. It didn't seem to matter that we were working at full capacity; our patients needed more than we could give. This wasn't about skill or dedication. It was strictly a numbers game. There were too many patients who required our help, and not enough hours in the day.

My patients were in need, but we didn't seem to have the proper structure in place that would allow them not only to survive but also to live the life they wanted. The death of Doyle had made that abundantly clear. That was a turning point for me, one that came with a lot of questions. What had Doyle needed that we couldn't give him? What could we have done differently that would have led to a better outcome? What had we missed? Those types of questions can prompt a spiral of *could haves* and *should haves* and *maybes* that can take anyone down. I've seen it happen, and it's tragic. My team had done their best, and it was up to me to learn from that—both for future patients and, in some way, to honor Doyle.

I took a step back and tried to evaluate the problem with a cool eye. What I saw was a team that was constantly falling short because it was lost in the details and burdens of daily practice. We worried about making room in the ICU for our patients, getting trained specialty nurses on the floor, working with anesthesia, building up the Cancer Center, meeting national guidelines, innovating, doing research, educating our patients. It was all too much. I made lists in the middle of the night because there were always too many things running through my brain for me to remain asleep. I hit the ground running every day, trying to put out fires but rarely having the time to even sit and think about my next step. I scarcely had enough time to make detailed rounds on all of my inpatients as I finished in the operating room at the end of the day. The needs of the patients came first, but they were overwhelming.

What could we do differently?

How could we serve our existing patients while still making room to treat new patients?

I turned to the people who supported me. All of us were spread so thin. They were loyal, hardworking, and talented. Surely together we could correct this inability to meet our patients' needs. So we talked. A lot. We talked about getting through patient visits faster so that we could add more appointment times. We even tried it. But that just led to more dissatisfaction. Because the truth is, rushing through a patient's session is worse than not seeing them at all.

Only when one day we noticed two patients animatedly sharing stories in the clinic waiting room did we edge closer to the solution. We knew these patients occasionally wanted advice from other patients as well as from me, so I had started connecting them to one another. I found the best person for them to talk to was someone who had been through the surgery. As we watched them conferring, supporting one another, Andrea and I caught each other's eye.

"Do you see what I see?" she asked, a smile forming on her face.

"Yes, I do," I responded.

We stood back and watched as they compared notes about their problems swallowing. Virtual strangers who likely wouldn't have had anything in common outside the hospital were talking like old friends, sharing how to make protein shakes, gain weight, and how to make broccoli cheese soup. They even shared their experiences

with queso, a popular local dish of melted cheese typically delivered to the mouth on a tortilla chip—only in this case, they drank
it straight from the bowl, a tasty way to gain weight. Some of the
suggestions they came up with sounded wild, and now and then I
thought they needed a moderator, someone knowledgeable who
could make sure people were not telling each other to do things
they shouldn't. Nevertheless, they were connecting on a fundamental level, with compassion, curiosity, and respect. They were able
to give each other more of what we were lacking, which was time.
More importantly, they were able to give each other something
we could never give them: the invaluable experience of talking to
someone who was walking the same path.

Little did we know it at the time, but that moment in the waiting
room planted the seed that would grow into the support group.
After that day in the clinic, Andrea and I started connecting more
patients to one another. I would meet someone who was having
a particular struggle and would say something to the effect of, "I
know a woman who is very much like you. In fact, she was in your
position about a year ago. She's doing so much better now and may
be able to help you." I'd reach out to the former patient and, with
her permission, would provide contact details so the two could
talk. It was medical matchmaking.

This is similar to the CanCare model, and it goes back to 1973,
when Anne Shaw Turnage, a wife and mother of three young children, was diagnosed with stage IV colon cancer. By all accounts a
formidable and spirited woman, she saw a profound lack of hope

among her fellow cancer patients. Believing that no one should face cancer alone, Anne sowed the seeds of support and encouragement that have become the hallmarks of CanCare, a Houston-based organization that, according to their website, trains cancer survivors to become caregivers, bringing "hope through survivorship to those with cancer and their caregivers."

The ideas were coming to me.

One idea that we put into operation was mentorship. As it works now, once patients have survived the worst part of their own illness, we offer them the opportunity to go through intensive training to learn how best to mentor others facing a new diagnosis of that illness. Not only does this provide the newly diagnosed with support informed by experience, but it also helps the survivor become more aware of how they navigated their own illness, moving past the fear and unknowns associated with a cancer diagnosis and finding a new sense of purpose in life. Serving as a mentor was also a healthy distraction from their own illness—it allowed them to take the focus off "I" and help others.

At the beginning we didn't provide any training to our former patients, but that didn't seem to be much of an impediment. And connecting people who were just beginning their cancer journey together with those who had recovered or were in remission really helped everyone. From there we looked at models such as Caring-Bridge, a digital platform whose mission is to "build bridges of care and communication providing love and support on a health journey." This wonderful resource underscored the need for connection and support, as did Gilda's Club, whose wise and inclusive motto is "Everyone's cancer is unique. Your support should be too." We looked at a lot of programs, some national and some local. While each of them brought great resources to our patients, none of them seemed to be exactly what we wanted. We needed something more. But it had to be simple. Plus, I wanted to be able to see what was happening and figure out how to spread myself more effectively around to the people I cared for.

Then it hit me.

When I was in high school, I had a friend who had a drinking problem. It was tough to see this smart young woman struggle so much in her recovery from alcoholism, but I knew I couldn't help her. At least not until she was ready to help herself. That day came when she asked me to go with her to an AA meeting. She just needed some moral support, she said, someone to help her get through the door and stay there. I only went to one meeting with my friend, but the experience stayed with me. I remembered the format and the atmosphere of respect and compassion as people got up to tell their stories. These sharing moments were profound, both for the person who was speaking and for the person who was listening. There was laughter. There were tears. Above all, there was acceptance.

That's what we needed. A support group where people dealing with cancer and its aftermath could come and talk openly about what they were going through. To acknowledge the inevitable, but also to thrive was the point. People could be positive or negative or anything in between, as long as they were real.

We started small. My secretary, Elaine, booked the hospital's conference room and invited all our current patients. Since nobody wants to do anything on a Monday, and since people get busier as the week goes on, we figured the first Tuesday of every month would be a good day. We even arranged to have our members' parking paid for by the hospital.

The first meeting consisted of about seven or eight people and was very awkward. Everyone stood around, not really knowing what to do or say. But there was a feeling of mutual curiosity and respect, and that was enough. We started small and grew. Watching the members connect with each other opened my eyes to the power of support. I could never have built the sort of relationship with them that they were developing with each other, nor did I want to interfere. Content to be a bystander, I spoke very little during those meetings. I didn't want to lead. I just wanted to see how it was all going to play out.

Elaine came to every single session. She listened closely to what everyone was saying, and as they talked about this issue or that, she or I would write it all down. A patient would talk about symptoms, severity, and frequency, and another would chime in to say, "Oh, yeah. That happened to me." We both sat up tall when we heard that. One person, for example, started to talk about vomiting frothy saliva every morning when she awoke, mentioning how gross it was. Her husband agreed. Someone else said the same thing happened to them, but they'd noticed that if they awoke a few times over the course of the night and drank water, it seemed to make the froth go away. Not only were they sharing problems, they were also sharing solutions.

Polly talked about how sometimes she could eat a meal without any problem, and then other times it would just come right back up. Stephen mentioned that his diarrhea got worse every time he ate sugar. The conversations started taking on a pattern: One person would say, "I have a problem . . ." Someone else would say, "I tried a few things to make it better, but the only thing that worked for me was . . ." Then the first person—and maybe someone else too—would say, "I'm going to try that!"

Not all of the problems brought up could be solved, but a lot of lessons were learned. And there was a bonus—a pretty big one at that. Because these exchanges showed me what my patients were struggling with, as well as their own makeshift remedies, I was able to apply my medical knowledge to their experience and come up with new solutions. For example, I learned that some people seem to be lactose intolerant after an esophagectomy. I had never read about that, nor had I recognized that it might be a problem. In fact, like most surgeons, I told my patients that after surgery they should rely on a liquid diet that was heavy on milk and milk-based protein shakes, which not only contained lactose but also had a lot of sugar. But the advice I was giving them was making some of them sick. Besides the lactose intolerance, others experienced what we call "dumping"—essentially low blood pressure, massive diarrhea, or feelings of extreme shakiness or sleepiness that can occur when a patient eats something sugary or high in carbohydrates. After I learned of these problems, I started coaching my patients to start with something called Muscle Milk. Easy to find at grocery stores and even gas stations, Muscle Milk isn't milk-based, nor does it contain a lot of sugar. It can be used in any recipe that calls for milk, and it's also high in protein.

Problem solved. At least one of them.

It didn't take long for us to realize the power of these Tuesday night meetings. After just a couple of sessions, Elaine and I saw how the support group was becoming a safe space for our patients to work things through honestly. This was where they could come when they needed a shoulder to cry on, when they needed someone to complain to. Somewhere they could hear another person say, "I'm sorry, friend. I know what that's like." That simple statement is a wonderful thing to hear whenever you are in a dark place.

Sometimes support came in the form of a strong cup of coffee and a bad joke. Other times it involved being given the space to vent. People in the group often spoke about their anger, frustration, and despair. Feeling powerless in the face of illness, these men and women just wanted to be heard. They wanted to be recognized as individuals, and they wanted acknowledgment of what they were going through, both for themselves as well as for the caregivers sitting next to them. It was validation they were after, and the support group provided that.

As for me, I thought the support group would be a good experiment, a way to meet the challenges of a busy practice. I had no idea that it would add to my life—or that it would bring me back to life. The support group offered me the same sense of purpose that I felt in surgery. It gave me that click that told me I was in the right place. That same glorious click that said, *This is where you belong.*

Five

The Fight of Their Lives

Jennifer was in her early twenties when she was diagnosed with synovial sarcoma, a type of soft-tissue sarcoma that had spread to her lungs. Synovial sarcoma can occur anywhere in the body, but almost always ends up in the lung—one of the body's many filters. Unfortunately, this gelatinous type of tumor is more difficult to remove than a solid mass, and it frequently causes pneumothorax, collapse of the lung. Otherwise healthy prior to her diagnosis, this vibrant young woman smiled easily and was unusually kind. I knew I shouldn't have identified with her, but I did. And we became close.

Having treated sarcoma patients while training at MD Anderson Cancer Center, I knew that those who had synovial sarcoma had the odds stacked against them. Chemotherapy isn't very effective, and the other treatment regimens we use are brutal, often causing patients to have terrible nausea, lose their hair, and suffer from anorexia. All this and most still succumb to the disease. It's a tragic pathway.

Early in my career, I noticed that few surgeons had an interest in treating sarcoma, which made me think that perhaps it might be a disease I could champion. It wasn't until I tried to secure funding to create a tissue bank that I realized why sarcoma is called an orphan disease.

According to the Centers for Disease Control and Prevention (CDC), about 264,000 women will be diagnosed with breast cancer every year. It's a highly visible cancer with tremendous support within the community. No one wants their mother or sister or daughter to die of this disease, so families are highly motivated to raise money to support research. And because that support and a large number of patients translates to dollars, drug companies are motivated to develop drugs to treat the condition. The second-leading cause of cancer death in women (lung cancer is number one), breast cancer death rates have been decreasing steadily over the last thirty years, for an overall decline of 43 percent, according to the American Cancer Society.[1] Better treatment is part of this, as is increased screening and awareness.

Sarcoma is an entirely different story. The infrequency of sarcoma (about thirteen thousand patients are diagnosed with soft-tissue sarcoma every year in the United States),[2] the predominantly young patient population, and the large variety of sarcoma subtypes make research and funding more complicated, resulting in fewer treatments with less cure. Treating patients with sarcoma can be frustrating for a surgeon. You feel like you're playing whack-a-mole as you pluck the tumors out of the lung knowing they're going to come right back.

Such was the case for Jennifer. When she came into the hospital, I remember taking her to the operating room for what appeared to be blood in the chest cavity. I started by inserting a small camera in the chest to try to figure out if I could drain the blood without doing a major thoracotomy (an incision over the side of the chest that includes cutting the muscle between the ribs and then cutting a rib and spreading the ribs apart with a crank). Her condition was unstable, with active bleeding, so she required a relatively urgent evaluation. There was no time for a multi-specialty discussion, extensive review of the growth rate of each tumor, meticulous counting of the number of lesions within the chest, or the possibility of chemotherapy to try to shrink the disease before operation.

Although we frequently have brief discussions with patients who present with urgent matters about end-of-life requests, palliative care, and hospice, when a young woman presents with active bleeding in the chest, going to the operating room seems like a reasonable plan. When I got into Jennifer's chest, it became clear that the small scope—the tiny camera I had inserted through a small incision in the hope that it would allow me to see what was going on—wouldn't do the job, so I performed a thoracotomy and explored. What I encountered was something I had never seen before: the gelatinous synovial sarcoma had taken over most of her left lung. What I was seeing wasn't just blood from a single ruptured tumor, but widely metastatic disease. There was really nothing I could do.

I called one of my senior professors from MD Anderson, and Dr. Garrett Walsh agreed that I should close. Trying to remove some or all of the lung in the circumstance would only result in further complications. I placed the necessary chest tubes, secured the ribs back to one another, closed the chest wall muscle back together in multiple layers, and then meticulously closed the skin like a plastic surgeon would, burying the absorbable sutures underneath the skin so that Jennifer would not have to come back to have any sutures removed.

After the surgery, we had long conversations when I made rounds. I found myself making extra time to sit at her bedside and talk with her. I pulled up a chair, and we had a lot of really difficult conversations. I ultimately discharged her from the hospital to go home on hospice. I called her medical oncologist, and they talked about different types of treatment options, most of which she had already exhausted. At the age of 38, Jennifer chose to go home and die.

I decided to visit her at home to see how things were going. Weeks after discharging her, I found her lying on the couch propped up on multiple pillows. She was wearing some faded blue jeans much like the ones I had on. The only problem was, hers seemed to have been placed on a skeleton, owing to the massive weight loss that had resulted since her discharge from the hospital. Her eyes were sunken and her temples were prominent, bulging above her eye sockets like architectural structures. Jennifer wasn't feeling well (that's an understatement), but still she garnered the energy to muster a smile.

I gave her a hug and we both started crying. I sat by her side, and we talked about life as if we were just two friends catching up. Jennifer's breathing was labored. I watched her chest rise and fall, and it became obvious that she was only using her right lung. The left side of her chest was still, failing to expand; it was likely filled with blood and tumors.

I came back by to see her several more times, and each time she was closer to death. For the first time in my life, I felt completely helpless. Most of the people who are referred to me for care have already been assessed by one or more other doctors and have a tumor that meets criteria for removal. Rarely do I have the opportunity to meet people who are beyond my help. Rarely do I have the opportunity to see people after I have performed surgery and there is nothing left to do. Most of these patients are now under the care of a medical oncologist or palliative medicine specialist. Palliative care doctors are the people who care for them around the time of death or who help cancer patients avoid suffering. These hero physicians watch people die every day. That's not something I can do. I know this, because watching the death of Jennifer haunts me to this day. Seeing her in her home changed me.

It is because of Jennifer's death—and the death of those like her—that I recommitted to treating sarcoma patients, studying the ablation of lung tumors (which are sometimes metastatic tumors from sarcoma primaries) and novel approaches for getting rid of these tumors inside the lung. Unfortunately, pharmaceutical companies are not financially incentivized to develop new treatments for patients with sarcoma. Developing effective drugs requires money and return on investment, and an expensive drug that will only be occasionally administered and that will only work on a small percentage of patients with a particular subtype of disease is not considered a financially viable endeavor. The worst part is that most of these sarcoma patients are children and young adults. With a focus on financial returns, drug companies tend to steer away from such rare diseases and instead focus on more prevalent cancers that affect more people. Better support for people with these less common diseases is desperately needed.

In my practice today, I still care for patients with sarcoma. Every time I see one on my patient list for the clinic, I flinch, recalling Jennifer—remembering her pain, knowing that sometimes all we can do is try to cut the thing out, hope they do better, and pray that some of the treatment works. Frequently we can help them get by for a while, a period in which they can fall in love, give back to the world, and spend a few more precious moments with family and loved ones. If only we could give them more time.

Michael Bradley didn't have much time. At least that was what his mother, Judy, worried about. And who could blame her? At twenty-three, Michael was one of my youngest esophageal cancer patients. I still remember the day I took him to the operating room for his esophagectomy. Judy was so distraught and distracted over her younger son undergoing surgery for one of the deadliest cancers in the world that she tripped and fell, hitting her head in the process. The poor woman had a black eye and a terrible bruise on her leg, as if *she* had just come out of surgery. Always good-natured despite the circumstances, Judy joked about the changing colors of her eye as it turned new shades of black, purple, and then green while Michael was in the hospital that week recovering from the surgery.

The selfless love of a mother for her children was a joy to witness. The rock of her family, Judy helped sustain her two sons (Michael's brother was going through a messy divorce) as they endured deep valleys of depression, anxiety, and misery. Because of the incredible support Judy gave to her children, they made it through their tribulations—Michael recovered and his brother got through his divorce and they both went on to enjoy happy marriages and have children of their own. And Judy became "Mimi" to her grandchildren, spreading the love to another generation of children.

Having enlisted in the military after high school, Michael had served two tours of duty in Iraq. He saw countless horrors, including the death of many of his comrades. Luckily, Michael made it home safely. There were aftereffects of the war, of course, such as the post-traumatic stress disorder (PTSD) that stayed with him for a very long time. But it would be another adversary that would bring him to me.

Upon returning to the States, Michael noticed he was having trouble swallowing, especially when he tried to eat bread or meat. This went on for about a month and seemed to be getting worse. One day he went over to his parents' house for lunch and suddenly started choking on a sandwich. He tried to drink some water, but the fluid came right back out of his mouth. His mother, Judy, ran over to help. When he gave the universal choking sign—grabbing his throat with both hands—Judy ran behind him and performed the Heimlich maneuver. Only when she squeezed his upper abdomen just below the breastbone, yelling at him to breathe, was Michael able to spit up the food and start breathing once again. Michael was relieved, exhausted, and scared. Judy was too. Michael then confessed to his family what had been going on. This was not the first time food had become stuck in his esophagus. Judy wasted no time calling their doctor, who got Michael scheduled for an endoscopy.

In almost all of the esophageal cancer patients I see, the disease does not get detected until the tumor is almost all the way through the wall of the esophagus and into the lymph nodes. Patients who have been experiencing symptoms of reflux, such as difficulty swallowing or serious heartburn and regurgitation, for five years are supposed to get an endoscopy, but most people don't know that. I'm not sure the majority of medical providers are even aware of that screening recommendation. This is why nearly everyone comes in with such advanced disease. Michael was lucky, as his disease was in an early stage. It was enough to make the food stick, but not bad enough to require chemotherapy. His general gastroenterologist knew immediately that it was cancer and sent him to a specialized interventional gastroenterologist, Dr. Isaac Raijman at Hermann Hospital in Houston, Texas, for removal of the cancer in another endoscopic procedure. Isaac was one of the "go-to" specialists for complicated procedures such as this.

Dr. Isaac Raijman was not just a colleague but also a friend. We both enjoyed painting, and our common love of good food and wine often found us having dinner together. The mutual respect we had for each other's talents at work made the relationship that much more rewarding. It was this friendship that led Isaac to call my cell phone while I was in my office at the clinic to tell me he was sending me someone stat. He'd found that the cancer could not be removed in an endoscopy and was going to require further surgery. Michael was so young, Isaac didn't want to give him the bad news and then have him wait a few weeks for an appointment to see a medical oncologist and a surgeon. He knew the family would have questions. He knew every minute without a plan would feel like a lifetime.

A number of clinics that specialize in breast care have tapped into a similar notion. Knowing that some women will require a follow-up ultrasound when they go in for a screening mammogram, they immediately send the patient for the ultrasound along with any subsequent testing that may be needed. This process ensures that no one goes home wondering, and I like it a lot. I liked it even more when I got to experience it firsthand with Michael, whom Isaac sent across the street to my clinic right after he finished the endoscopy.

Michael's mom, Judy, was with him—exactly where she would remain throughout the entire journey. Her love for her son was boundless and intense. That was the first thing I saw when I met them. Judy was always touching Michael, staying physically in contact with him as if to keep him from floating away. Michael's father arrived shortly after; Judy had called him to join them after hearing the news. Though at our first meeting I thought he might have been in the military as well, I later discovered he was actually an attorney, with a major role in running the regional federal district court system. A man of few words, he chose those words carefully, and of the three of them, he was always the last to ask questions. We talked about basic details of cancer—how we would make sure the tumor had not spread to the abdominal cavity, getting a feeding tube in, ensuring that he was getting adequate nutrition to optimize his chances of having a good recovery, and what kinds of complications to expect.

I couldn't get over how healthy Michael looked. His muscular form, perfect posture, bright eyes, and handsome smile were all hindering me from focusing on how sick he was on the inside. It simply didn't make sense. Just one week prior another young man from the military had been referred to me with the same diagnosis—though he had stage IV disease, which would lead to his death within six months. When I thought about it, I realized that Michael was the fourth military patient I had either seen or heard of who was diagnosed with esophageal cancer at a young age. There were also some rumors that many young men were coming back from Iraq with other strange cancers. I made a mental note to check into this.

Michael simply asked me point-blank, "How long do I have?" I told him I wasn't sure, but we would have a much better idea once we got the final pathology report back after surgery. Things become much more predictable once we are able to see more than the tip of the iceberg. Judy wanted to know how difficult the surgery was and what they needed to do to get him ready for it. She wanted to know how many people had had the surgery and the percentage who died from the operation itself. I gave her the statistics and told her that most people have some type of complication during their initial recovery period, and many often struggle with symptoms even afterward. I also shared with her specific data on how many of these surgeries I performed on average every year, along with alternatives to surgery. Her questions were many, but it was clear to me they weren't going to remember a word I said past "You have cancer" and "You need surgery." That is all most people ever recall from that first appointment.

Because I know patients are hardly ever able to remember these things, I built a website offering patient education materials for them. The internet as a whole is too scary, and most of the information that comes up only deals with how "average" patients do, which is not good. I also made an hour-long video that covers the information I present in that initial visit, allowing them to go back over it later, after the initial shock of the cancer diagnosis has passed. I realized this was necessary after having the same conversations over and over again, patient after patient. They get home after the initial visit and their families have so many questions, and at that point they are still trying to get past the "you have cancer" part. They need all of the resources they can get to tell them what is to come.

I'd given many diagnoses over the years; had given bad news to innumerable patients. This one hurt more than usual. Michael had come in thinking his whole life was ahead of him. I couldn't believe it. Neither could he. He was in perfect health otherwise and seemed to be the kind of man who could fight anything. We spent time talking about the diagnosis and how it would change his life. I purposely steered him away from discussing a prognosis because I wanted him to feel optimistic and stay strong as he braced for the biggest fight of his life.

"I don't remember ever having reflux," was all Michael could say. He felt like he had done something wrong or maybe had missed something. I emphasized that this surprises everyone when it happens. I tried to reassure him because the disease looked to be in an early stage, and I pointed out that it could be considered encouraging that he didn't have to go through chemo and radiation therapy. I didn't mention the other cases of this cancer I had seen and heard about in the other soldiers who had been in Iraq; that would have been cruel, and life had been cruel enough. And, as it turned out, his experience in Iraq would complicate his struggle in other ways. The day I did Michael's esophagectomy, he awoke from anesthesia thinking he was in battle again. So strong was this belief that he actually tried to kill my PA, Andrea, as he emerged from the gas. Strapped to the bed, hearing people shouting at him to settle down, Michael thought he was being held hostage. He struggled violently and tried to fight the OR team, still with a breathing tube in his throat. Three men had to hold him down to keep him from hurting Andrea.

Despite his muscular strength and despite being trained to kill, Michael was actually a gentle soul suffering with PTSD. The trauma that Michael had experienced when he was in Iraq had come crashing down on him, activating his fight-or-flight response. That's how it works. When he learned afterward what had happened as he was coming out of the anesthesia, he apologized profusely to Andrea. Clearly, he had no memory of the event. She understood that he wasn't responsible for the terror that coursed through him. She was gracious, kind, and forgiving, as always. I wondered if this new journey might give him an even worse case of PTSD. War and now cancer—which battle was more harrowing?

A little while after surgery, Michael attended a meeting of the support group, accompanied by his mother. I think she was the one who made him come. Judy was incredible. As I would learn throughout the years, she was full of love for everyone, the kind of person who holds everyone else up. Years after I left Houston, she would text me pictures of Michael and his family or a blessing, like "Every minute God cares for you" (based on 1 Peter 5:7), and "Because every second He loves you" (Jeremiah 31:3). Sometimes she would send a recipe. She was always present somewhere in my mind, and I always smiled whenever I thought of how much she cared for and helped her sons.

Supporting her son at every turn, Judy shared stories of how brave he was, and how kind. She even tried some matchmaking for him to provide a distraction. Judy made sure Michael was eating well, getting exercise, and feeling the love every second of the day. But she didn't provide that support blindly. There were many times when Judy called out her son for being less than honest. I remember one support group meeting when someone asked Michael how he was doing and he said, "Oh, sure, yeah. I'm doing fine."

Well, his mother had something to say about that. "No, you are not fine. You are a long way from being fine."

Michael looked like a little boy who had been caught with a fistful of cookies. He shifted his glance to the floor, unable to meet his mother's eyes.

"I found him sitting on the counter the other night, shoveling sugar into his mouth," Judy said.

I turned to Michael and asked him in front of the group what was happening. He replied, "I felt this burning sensation come up into my throat, and green stuff started coming back up, and I couldn't drink enough water to kill the burning pain. Shoving sugar down my mouth seemed like the only way to get it to stop." Patients often tell me that phenomenon, called bile reflux, is the worst thing in the world.

Because of the memory of that moment, I have completely changed the way I do surgery. I was taught to cut the emptying valve from the stomach, the pylorus, to allow the stomach tube to empty better. My older professors told me I had to do this in spite of the lack of clear evidence that it was the right thing to do. In fact, it occurred to me that a lot of our practice and techniques were based not on measuring patient-reported outcomes but rather on what the surgeon thought was best. We needed better data. After going to China and seeing that they don't cut the pylorus during esophagectomy anymore, I realized that the dogma I'd been taught might be wrong. I started to question all the technical decisions we make in the operating room and how they affect each patient. I haven't cut a pylorus at the time of esophagectomy in over fifteen years. Now I inject Botox into the valve to temporarily paralyze the muscle during the period after surgery, which also allows the stomach tube to empty effectively. This lasts for about five months, and then it wears off, encouraging the valve to tighten back up just enough to keep the bile reflux from happening. Now I rarely have a patient complain of bile reflux like Michael did that day.

When I heard Michael describe his symptoms that day in the support group, I knew something was wrong. I insisted on seeing him in the clinic the next week and made him get more scans and a swallow study. I found that part of his intestine had herniated above the diaphragm, creating an opening where the new stomach tube was. Called a para-conduit hernia, this happens more often when people have a minimally invasive esophagectomy, since there is so little scar tissue to hold things in place. The real problem with these hernias is that the symptoms are often so subtle that people don't know they have them. No wonder Michael was suffering. Once again, Judy's intervention had made a difference.

I couldn't help but wonder what would have happened to Michael without the support group, without his mother sitting behind him urging him to speak the truth. We might have gone a long time without knowing what was happening. Thank goodness we were able to fix it. Thank goodness I was able to hear about how the bile reflux affected him. I changed my practice because of what I was learning. We were all benefiting.

Caregiving matters. Caregivers matter.

As I said, Michael was the fourth young soldier I had seen or heard of with esophageal cancer in a six-month time frame. I decided to call the Veterans Administration to see if there might be some common thread, but to no avail. Gaining access to military records or initiating a query into cancer-related outcomes from potential exposures such as burn pits is difficult. The military healthcare system does not welcome outsiders or allow them to learn much at all.

Watching Michael go through the rest of his life is one of the greatest gifts I have ever received. Staying in touch with his mother is another. I love seeing how he has enjoyed such a life made possible by the mere fact that we took the cancer out and later fixed a problem. That procedure helped Michael turn a corner. He went on to run a marathon, marry, father two beautiful girls, and have a wonderful life. Judy once sent me a picture of Michael standing with his family, a huge smile on his face. She wrote in a note that he wouldn't be here if it wasn't for us. Well, that made me ugly-cry. I cried for what he had endured, for those in the support group we had lost, for the presence of cancer, for the things I wished I had done better for my patients, and for all the pain that sometimes seems to rot us from the inside.

Today, Michael is fourteen years out from his diagnosis, in that rare place in a cancer journey where we use the word "cure." He asked me if he needed to continue to get endoscopies, or if he needed CT scans to monitor whether the cancer might have returned. Although that can happen once in a blue moon for someone who has been free of cancer for so long, I told him it was unlikely. I gave him some things to watch for, like more swallowing problems, unexplained weight loss, excessive fatigue, or bleeding from anywhere, and that if he experienced any of those changes he should get an endoscopy or a scan. He still sleeps with the head of his bed at an incline, and about once a month feels some reflux happening; when that happens, he'll occasionally get up in the middle of the night to walk around to get things to settle down once again. Overall, the quality of his life is good. Most days he forgets he ever had cancer or an esophagectomy.

And that is a beautiful thing to hear.

Six

A Village of Support

There are many different kinds of patient caregivers. They exist within medical institutions, within the community at large, even within our own homes. *Especially* within our homes. In my position as a surgeon, I have been privileged to witness a variety of levels of care, from the assistance provided to homeless patients without family or resources to that given to royalty who have an entire army of personal physicians and attendants as well as family. Support beyond measure.

A committed ally can make all the difference in a patient's recovery. There's no way to overestimate the practical or emotional support that a good caregiver can provide. On the whole, people who have a partner in care, someone to stay by their side through the ups and downs of treatment, not to mention help them navigate our healthcare system, do far better than those who don't. Which is why when I set up the support group, I recommended patients come with their caregivers. It was one of the most important things I did.

Bringing caregivers to a support group provides them with a network of their own while allowing them to see and be inspired by how others are giving and receiving support. Just being able to connect with people in a similar position, to share information and perhaps a strong shoulder . . . well, that's just about everything. As for the patients themselves, they report back the benefits of having their caregivers attend, which includes finally being able to acknowledge clear symptoms and problems (something the patients may have been reluctant to do), being able to discuss the impact of complications (something patients and their caregivers might not have understood), and finding even more ways to encourage each other as their "village of support" grows (something patients and their caregivers all needed).

In basic terms, a patient caregiver is someone who tends to the needs or concerns of a person requiring assistance because of limitations incurred due to illness, injury, or disability. They may aid with health and social needs, as well as the general aspects of daily living, such as bathing and dressing, shopping, paying bills, and providing transportation. And let's not forget the emotional sustenance that goes along with helping someone who is being treated for an illness.

Most of these patient caregivers are family members, but—as we know now more than ever—family can be by choice rather than related by blood. My favorite family-by-choice story is that of Dr. Andrea Wolfe, a thoracic surgeon and colleague who works in New York City. Andrea was a resident in the neonatal intensive care unit

(NICU) when a mother abandoned her special-needs infant, born with complex medical issues. Seeing this vulnerable child all alone, without a parent to comfort him, Andrea crossed a line and held him herself. She grew to love the baby—it didn't take long—and eventually adopted him. Today, she continues to care for him. They are family.

A lot closer to home, I have become one of the medical caregivers for my stepfather. Despite the fact that he has a new wife and four children, when he had a stroke this last winter I was one of the first to be called. I organized the healthcare team to make important decisions around his medication, activity, rehabilitation, and just generally meeting his needs. As his medical power of attorney, I have helped him optimize his health and weighed in on choices that can have a lifetime of consequences, such as navigating complicated issues with chronic pain, spinal injury, atrial fibrillation, and gastrointestinal bleeding. Because I am a physician, much of this responsibility falls naturally onto my shoulders, a duty I take on happily. I know very well that if one member of my family becomes ill, my phone will be the first to ring. I'm okay with that. In fact, I count on it.

I'm inspired by the caregivers I get to witness every day, by the family, friends, community members, and clergy who accompany patients to the clinic, supporting them through some of the toughest days of their lives.

The ones who impress me most are those who care for patients they may not even be related to. Beverly Schorre was one such person. A woman of faith who practiced what she preached, Beverly routinely volunteered to take people to medical appointments, visit them at home, make sure they had food, and check on them when they had no one. She expected nothing in return.

I met Beverly at First Presbyterian in Houston. A wonderful old church, the first iteration of which was built in the mid-nineteenth century and lit by whale-oil lamps, it was a warm and close community. I took my children with me to First Presbyterian. My in-laws also attended, as did many of my colleagues. As did Polly.

An actress when she was younger, Polly had been a nanny for a friend of mine who had previously lived on our street in Houston. When the family moved away, Polly would have been alone, if not for the warm and supportive community of the church. Beverly and Polly were stalwarts of First Presbyterian. Friends with a common purpose, they knew and respected each other. And yet the depth of their bond did not truly develop until one needed the other. Before that, it was more cordial, superficial, and polite. It wasn't until Polly became ill and Beverly escorted her to appointments and to the support group that they learned to be unguarded with one another. Being unguarded—this is what I call being comfortable enough to be weird, yourself, and real. You can recognize it when you see it. No one is trying to impress anyone else. Trust is present and unconditional love is there to stay.

During the time I ran the support group, I can barely remember ever having a single meeting without Beverly and Polly being present, until Polly's condition deteriorated and she died. I truly believe the support she received from Beverly helped her make it to the point where she was cured from the esophageal cancer. With Beverly's help, Polly not only survived surgery but thrived.

It wasn't always easy. Polly was bitter at times. She was angry at her cancer. A lifetime of smoking led to chronic obstructive pulmonary disease (COPD) and had left her bound to a large oxygen tank, and she missed the spontaneous person she used to be. Polly hated living in an assisted living facility so far away from the rest of the world, and she missed the old friends who had died years before her. Still, she was truly grateful for the selfless care and love shown to her by Beverly. Most of the time Beverly sat behind Polly at the support group, remaining quiet. However, there were times when Beverly would encourage Polly to become more vulnerable, or to be more or less vocal as the situation required. When Polly would roll her eyes at a comment made by one of the newer survivors who was still learning how to describe their symptoms, Beverly would place her hand on Polly's shoulder and whisper something wise, calm her down, or ask her to explain to the group why she was so grumpy. Perhaps Polly was acting out because of the loss of another friend. Perhaps the topic of children had come up in the group, and she was regretting the fact that she never had children. But it was Beverly who always got Polly to soften up and open up.

Beverly also knew how important the support group meetings were to Polly and would have made sure she was there even if she had to bring her on a stretcher.

Over the years, Beverly and Polly became more than caregiver and patient. They became best friends. Beverly brought Polly to my daughter's dedication when she was born. Looking like great-aunties, they rushed across the vestibule to greet the small child in my arms. For nine months they had watched her grow in my belly during support group. Polly acted like Grace was her own grandchild. The way she touched Grace was as if this child was the most precious thing in the world (which to me she was). I have a cherished photo from that day, and whenever I am sad or feeling overwhelmed by the weight of my job, I turn to that moment and remember the good.

Polly died four months after that. Beverly spoke at her funeral. She talked about Polly's grace and humor, and about her sometimes crusty disposition. She spoke with honesty and love. Polly may have cursed like a sailor, but her faith was deep. She loved God and was happy to tell anyone about it.

I carry a tremendous amount of guilt with me because Polly died shortly after I announced my intent to move to Rochester to work at Mayo Clinic. No one knows what tethers us to earth, but it's safe to say those things Polly loved were slowly being taken away from her one by one until she might have felt it was time. I sometimes feel like perhaps Polly hung on so that she could finally meet Grace, and then felt like she could let go. I also wonder if she felt my move would mean the end of the support group she leaned on so much. We were her tribe. I will never have a day go by that I don't miss her. After Polly died, Beverly gave me a small nativity pin that was one of Polly's most precious items. There was no obligation. There was no blood relationship. There was just service, sacrifice, and love. Family by choice.

It was Rosalyn Carter who wisely said, "There are only four kinds of people in the world. Those who have been caregivers. Those who are currently caregivers. Those who will be caregivers, and those who will need a caregiver." Unfortunately, even with that acknowledgment, we don't do enough to care for caregivers. The selfless act of looking after another person can be detrimental to a caregiver who ignores their own health and well-being at the expense of their loved one. According to the CDC:

> Caregiving is an increasingly common experience in middle and older adults that cuts across demographic groups. The need for caregivers is expected to grow due to the continued increases in the older adult population. Many middle-aged and older adults who are not currently caregivers do expect to provide care in the future. People are caregivers for various amounts of time, but most people provide care for six months or more and for many it is equivalent

to a part-time job. These caregivers may have a substantial burden of disability and chronic disease as they care for others.[1]

It's well documented that caregivers may ignore their own health while taking such good care of others. Catering to the lives of those they love, they discount any indication that all might not be well within themselves. A 2011 national health and aging trend study[2] and national study of caregiving found that there were an estimated 14.9 million caregivers assisting 7.6 million care recipients. More than half of caregivers reported a burden related to caregiving, meaning they suffered physical, emotional, or financial hardships.

When researchers weighed all the variables, they found that caregivers who assisted with instrumental activities of daily living, health management tasks, and health system logistics were more likely to experience burden, as were female caregivers, adult child caregivers, caregivers in poor health, caregivers with anxiety symptoms, and those using respite care.[3]

I always try to tell caregivers to plan to care for themselves, to stay connected to resources that provide relief, so they don't become burned out. I also tell them to accept help when it's offered, because as time goes by, people lose enthusiasm to help. This is a marathon and not a sprint. Caregivers need support to make sure they take care of themselves. Many become so wrapped up in caring for their loved one with a chronic illness that they neglect friendships, their own health, finances, and many other things healthy individuals have the luxury of attending to on a regular basis. Just as cancer patients need someone to step in and offer help, so do their caregivers. General offers of help, while they may be well-meaning, don't really do much to lift the caregiver's burden. Specific suggestions, such as "Can I pick up anything for you at the grocery store?" or "Can I come over Wednesday afternoon to give you a break?" are much more helpful and much more likely to be accepted. And never forget the power of a strong shoulder or a listening ear. Being there for a caregiver—just as they are there for the person being cared for—can mean everything. It's just a matter of showing up.

The support group has taught me one thing: build your village. We are all social animals, and we cannot survive alone. The caregivers in our support group learned this, just as they learned to lean on one another. It wasn't easy at first. So used to looking after others, to being the strong shoulder for their loved ones suffering from cancer, they were reluctant to show any vulnerability. It can be hard to dismantle that tough, can-do attitude. But like the people they were looking after, these caregivers also found strength in numbers and in sharing. It wasn't just recipes and solutions they shared; it was stories. They talked about how tired they were, how they felt frustrated, frightened, and sometimes just plain annoyed. And they shared their successes too.

Caregiving can be isolating, and the feeling that you're at someone's beck and call can really wear you down to the point that you have little left for yourself. That's probably why caregivers seemed to enjoy coming to the support group just as much as the patients did.

And the group sessions made them feel less alone when they were experiencing the overwhelming stress of waiting for surveillance scans to come back. Waiting for news—good or bad—feels a little easier when you have someone there with you. Many caregivers felt like they were always waiting for the other shoe to drop.

That's why we started finding reasons to celebrate. We celebrated birthdays, anniversaries, births—just about everything but Groundhog Day. When I saw the joy these celebrations brought, we then got the idea to start celebrating five years of survival with a "cure" party. Pronouncing someone cured from esophageal cancer is a rare and wonderful thing, and it calls for the best of all celebrations, for the patient and for the caregiver. Although some patients got to ring a bell at the end of their treatment, they needed more. These parties represented resilience and survival. They represented summiting a mountain as big as Mount Everest, with a similar death rate within that first thirty days. They were a moment to exhale, to let the fear go and move on. As we celebrated the survival of Polly, Stephen, and John, we saw the joy magnified within the group, especially for the caregivers who felt the lifting of a weight. Now they were back on an even playing field with their loved ones, back to a place where they could take care of one another, where support was—once more—a mutual thing.

Seven

Just Like Family

John and Juanita were one of those couples out of the introductory scene of *When Harry Met Sally*. They completed each other's sentences, one correcting the other on important details. "It was a Wednesday," John would say. "No," Juanita would counter. "It was a Tuesday. I know because we were waiting for the lottery numbers to be drawn." They shared the same jokes, each trying to beat the other to the punch line. And they asked dozens of questions. It was hard to remember John was the one with cancer, since Juanita was so involved in the conversations. "Dr. Blackmon, is it true that people can get leg swelling after a vagotomy?"

Juanita wasn't the only involved caregiver, however. Others asked me questions like:

"Why is everyone telling me to drink my liquids at a different time than when I eat? How am I supposed to wash all this food down?"

"What do you think about that new medication advertised on TV? The one where they're all riding bikes and eating salad? Is that something that might help me?"

John and Juanita loved to talk. And Stephen and Polly, other patients participating in the group, resented them for it. The Juanita-Polly-Stephen war was waged at every meeting. You could count on it just like you could count on the Texas Medical Center to flood every time it rained for more than an hour straight. Sometimes it was funny and sometimes it was scary. At times it was almost entertaining—if you took out the part about how this was a support group centered around helping cancer survivors. There were a lot of emotions roiling around that room.

For example, Juanita would start talking about John's blood sugar going low, and Stephen and Polly would roll their eyes. Sometimes Polly would blurt out, "For God's sake, Juanita, let someone else talk!" At that point, the newer group members would look on slack-jawed, shocked by the raw anger. Others—those who were more accustomed to the bickering—would smile nervously, laugh it off, or glance the other way. *Nothing to see here, folks. Just our friends going at each other . . . again.* It was a fact of life. Just as siblings fight in the backseat of the car, our members quarreled in the support group meetings. I guess it was to be expected. This was, after all, a family of sorts.

And just like family, we laughed together and cried together. We held each other up. Sure, there was fighting, but there was also friendship, and even dating. Patterns evolved too. Some members liked to sit close to one another, align within groups, and form close friendships. Typically, the more seasoned members sat at one end of the room while the newer participants tended to sit at the other.

This likely happened because the space would fill from the back of the room to the front, with long-timers coming early to socialize with friends and catch up before the meeting started. Sometimes a member might bring esophagectomy-friendly snacks, like mashed potatoes, sugar-free pudding cups, or peanut butter bites, or we might invite a guest speaker, usually an expert on a particular topic people were struggling with.

Yet, as much as the meetings were always worthwhile, they could be challenging at times. The whole purpose of a support group is for patients and their families to voice their concerns, to understand that they're not alone, and perhaps to share ways of coping with their diagnosis and its aftermath. But these groups can be as complicated as the people who attend them. Nobody expects smiles and warm hugs all the time. It's only natural that there will be friction and the occasional clash of personalities or viewpoints. But that's just at the surface. Real support—the kind that can get you through the most troubled times—goes deep and transcends personal preferences. Support isn't about simple likes and dislikes, about who votes for whom, or who went to this college or that one. It's about caring for another person in a meaningful way. It's about respecting what someone else is going through and being there for it all.

Time and again I saw members become brave enough to speak about the discomfort of their symptoms, the difficulty in coping, and sometimes just plain loneliness. These moments of admission were tremendous. By confessing to a group of people who listened with care and compassion, members were able to normalize their

suffering to some degree. That alone went a long way toward al-
leviating feelings of isolation. Not to mention that one person's
experiences made it possible for others to share theirs. There really
is strength in numbers.

Sharing in front of a group isn't always easy, but it can be
invaluable..

I'm used to having tough conversations with my patients. I tell
them what they need to do for the good of their health and hope
that they do it. Notice I said "hope." Not everyone takes my advice.
Doyle certainly never did, and he suffered severe consequences as a
result. There are so many reasons a patient may not follow doctor's
orders. It's hard for me to accept this, knowing as I do that people
who don't adhere to their treatment plan are more likely to experience complications and disease progression. I do my best to let
my patients know why a particular course of action is advisable and
ask them if there's anything in their lives that might get in the way of
following it, but sometimes that's not enough. There are many barriers
to adherence: There may be language issues or financial obstacles,
patient depression, or stress. Not to mention stubbornness. People
who were stubborn before their diagnosis aren't magically going to
change. Old dogs like Doyle do not like to learn new tricks.

Sometimes, however, what a doctor can't achieve, another patient can. A person who has trouble remembering to take his meds
might be told by another to set an alarm. I recall one woman who
told another member that she takes her evening medication at the
same time every day, when *Jeopardy* comes on. "It's a cue for me,"

she told him. "The minute the music comes on for Final Jeopardy, I know it's time." Another group member, an older man, mentioned that he didn't always remember what his doctor told him. That's a common problem, and more than a few members offered up suggestions. "Ask the doctor if you can record the session on your phone," one recommended. "Write things down when you're still in the examining room," another said. "Do what I do," advised a third. "Get your doctor to slow down. Say you know she's busy, but if she takes a few minutes longer with this visit, you may not need to come back so many times. That always gets 'em!"

Dealing with issues head-on can be hard, but it seems to happen organically within the group. "You have to accept your bad days just like you've had to accept your diagnosis," I remember one member telling another. That's not something that people want to hear from their doctors, but hearing it from another cancer patient, someone who is dealing with what you're dealing with, feels profound. The internet is chock-full of recommendations for the cancer patient: *Get a second opinion. Make time for self-care. Be kind to yourself. Prioritize responsibilities. Stay connected.* Sure, nobody would argue with this advice. But most people would prefer to have it come from an empathetic person who knows firsthand what they are facing rather than read a bulleted list on yet another website. The give-and-take that arises from the meetings is immeasurable. And not just from patients, but caregivers too.

I have to confess that one of my favorite moments occurs when a patient is talking about something they do and then gets corrected by their caregiver with a loud "You don't do that!" The caregiver will call the group member out on their behavior much the same way my husband does when I talk about "being a runner." I haven't been running for over a year now, but I still like to call myself a runner.

Caregivers who acknowledge a patient's struggles are vital in helping them course correct, mostly by keeping them honest. It's one thing to hide the truth from yourself; it's quite another to hide it from your caregiver and your support group. Time and time again I've seen caregivers tease out a more truthful or expanded story simply by raising an eyebrow or asking gently, "Are you telling us *everything*?" Once prompted—well, sometimes it takes more than one prompt—members are able to come clean and open up about what they've been dealing with, the good, the bad, and the embarrassing.

Solutions and support. That's the value of the support group. By acknowledging struggles, a support group can provide answers and promote positivity. But it's not a straight line from here to there. Sometimes in order to get to the positive we need to wade through the negative, to confront it. Often newcomers are still struggling with grief and disbelief. Some worry about being stigmatized by people they don't know. Others even feel some guilt. They should have quit smoking. They should have eaten better foods or exercised more. They should have done this. They should have done that. A cancer diagnosis is met with dozens of these *should haves*. Having the opportunity to discuss these feelings with others is invaluable, especially for those who are reluctant to share details of their illness.

It's never easy to hear the words "You have cancer." Some people avoid talking about their illness because they don't want to worry the ones they love. Others don't want to be looked at differently and they certainly don't want to be treated as a patient. "With some people, you can just tell they're on edge. Like, you can see them wondering how much longer I'm going to be around," said one annoyed group member. Another talked about the clumsy response he got when he shared his diagnosis: "A guy at work said, 'The survival rate for your cancer is really low. You must be worried.' As if I didn't know how to Google that myself. As if I actually *wanted* that information." Everyone groaned at the phrase "Let me know if you need anything." People mean well, but the fact is, nobody really responds to that kind of offer. "I just can't with the *anything*," one vocal member said. "Offer to cut my grass or pick up some chicken soup. Tell me you'll walk my dog. But offering *anything* is the same as offering *nothing*."

The support group reminded people they weren't alone. Being in a place where they could witness other people's struggles, where they could gain tools to fight specific problems, coping strategies, and caregiver support, gave them courage. The friendships sustained them. The promise of knowing they could return and be understood gave the patients confidence to go out in the world feeling sustained. As Robert Frost said, "The best way out is always through."

Eight

See the Matrix

The support group had been going for a few years when Maureen joined us. She'd had a gastrectomy (removal of the stomach) and a partial esophagectomy. I felt it was important to include other patients who'd undergone gastrectomies, since that was part of my practice, as it is for many thoracic surgeons.

Caring for gastrectomy patients is very similar to caring for esophagectomy patients. Because the esophagus and stomach are so close to each other, removing either of them will result in a very similar manifestation of symptoms, problems, and complications. Maureen's tumor was primarily centered around the stomach area, so she still had a large part of her esophagus. Nevertheless, the surgery caused a significant drop in her weight, something she continues to struggle with some fifteen years after her cure.

An attractive woman in her mid-sixties who came regularly to the support group, Maureen was a uniformly positive person who liked to talk about her grandchildren, Texas football games, and her love of travel. She always had nice things to say to the other members, and as a teacher, she was really good at having discussions with numerous people at once. ("Crowd control," as I thought of it some days.) Maureen taught me a lot about creating consistency, about keeping the room safe for everyone to feel like they could speak, and about the importance of hearing from even the quietest voices. Empathetic, kind, and a very good listener, she was particularly helpful in drawing out some of the shy members. You could always count on her to make them feel more comfortable.

Maureen had been a teacher in a small Jewish school in Houston. She clearly loved her profession and talking about her students, of whom there were many. I shouldn't have been surprised when one crossed her path at the hospital, but I was. At the time, I was having difficulty getting surgical residents to spend time in the clinic. Everyone has parts of the job that they love and parts of the job that they dread. This is as true for a plumber or a teacher as it is for a surgeon. That being said, I don't know any surgeons who dread going into the operating room. Everything just clicks into place the moment you walk into the OR. MRIs show that the part of your brain that is synced up with what you do and where you find your joy, with how you define yourself—all those automatic things that go into making sense of the world around you—lights up when you are doing those things.

Many young surgeons consider the OR the place where they make a difference. What they don't seem to realize is the value of the work done *before* surgery. A great part of a patient's outcome is determined in the clinic. When we first get a patient who isn't eating and has lost a lot of weight, we have to either place a feeding tube or send them to a nutritionist to make sure that they find ways to put that weight on and keep themselves from becoming severely deconditioned. Interrupting that downward spiral makes all the difference. Patients who have multiple medical issues and present with all of them getting worse at the same time need a complex medical system to look at all the individual problems and try to resolve them in order to make them better candidates for surgery: the selection of patients is one of the most important things. Patient selection is one of the main focus points of our oral board exam we administer to certify a surgeon as safe and competent to practice their specialty. Being able to recognize who can benefit from surgery right away, who needs to improve some aspects of their health in order to be able to benefit from surgery, and who is unlikely to ever be a good candidate for surgery is both an art and a skill. This is where the wisdom comes in. It cannot be easily understood from reading a textbook. Good patient selection comes from experience and exposure. Equally important is setting expectations for those patients who are at high risk of complications, as many patients would prefer to have the opportunity to select the path for themselves knowing the risk that is involved. Setting expectations, evaluating risk, making the decision to operate (or not), obtaining consent, performing a good assessment of health, collecting a good history, and communicating are all things that happen in the clinic *before* surgery. Together, these are the foundation of what we must teach our residents and the fellows who train under us.

Today, these things have to happen typically within a thirty-minute clinic visit or less. This nearly impossible task can be accomplished only with either a team approach or the help of a systematic checklist that prevents things from falling through the cracks. Learning to create, follow, and build teams around these care pathways and develop good decision-making is one of the most important skills a surgeon will learn during their training. Not to mention that sound decision-making is fundamental to achieving board certification, and that the best way to learn how to decide when to operate, and when not to, is by being in the clinic.

Sadly, these days almost no residents follow patients longitudinally—that is, over the course of their treatment and afterward. Back when I was in training, when we residents worked over a hundred hours a week, we would have more of a relationship with patients because we'd stay in one hospital on one particular service and see them throughout the entire course of their care. Changes to the structure of residencies mean that now when patients come back for follow-up after their surgery, most residents have rotated off that particular service and are on to another experience, like colorectal surgery or cardiac surgery or a completely different program altogether. Instead of the old apprenticeship model, where young doctors might be aligned with a practice for years at a time, giving them the chance to witness the evolution of both patient care and the patient relationship, the experience now consists of short intervals in a variety of practices. That means most of their experience is centered around surgery and post-operative care.

Occasionally a resident may see a patient in the clinic before or after surgery, but it's relatively rare that this will be someone they will operate on or have operated on.

I often thought one of the best things a resident training program could do is assign each resident a few patients to monitor for an extended period of time. That type of follow-up would demonstrate to the residents the longitudinal effects of the surgeries they perform or participate in. I couldn't do that, alas, but I could mandate that my residents attend the support group. The idea here was for them to connect with survivors at different points after surgery. I believed it was the best way, perhaps the only way, for these young doctors to understand the effects of surgery—physical, emotional, social, and relational.

There's nothing like being able to interact with a patient to see the impact of a single surgery on all aspects of a patient's life over time. Being in a less formal setting like a support group emboldens patients to speak more openly about their struggles, allowing these residents to understand the impact of that surgery for a patient. They could also witness—perhaps for the first time—the wonderful things that occur when one patient helps another. Giving the residents the ability to see how we all cared for and supported one another was a unique and special gift. I found that most of my residents had some kind of transformation because of the support group. They certainly were more humane and caring in the way they talked about the people they treated. Instead of referring to someone primarily in terms of a diagnosis, such as "a seventy-year-old man with hypertension and cancer," residents started using names, personalizing histories, and using introductions like "A very pleasant seventy-year-old man named Jack, who works as a farmer, has three children, and loves surfing and listening to the Beach Boys, presents with hypertension and cancer." Most of the residents told me that their experience with the support group made them better physicians and surgeons.

And then there was Yoav. I remember the first time he entered the meeting room and the absolute delight when Maureen recognized him as one of her former students. She was so delighted with all he had accomplished and, like a proud teacher, introduced him to everyone in the group. "I knew he'd end up doing big things," she told everyone. Yoav was thrilled to reconnect with his old teacher, although sorry to hear about her health struggles. But this put a whole new spin on things for him.

Much like Neo, the protagonist from *The Matrix,* Yoav was finally able to "see the matrix." Meaning he was able to understand the complexity of these patients' lives. He knew from his training that a feeding jejunostomy tube (a small tube that passes through the abdominal wall and into the small bowel) is needed for patients who aren't healthy enough to eat anything by mouth, and that the feeding utilized a pump to push the food into their bodies. What he didn't know—at least not until he heard it at the support group—was that this meant chronic pain around the insertion site, as well as a myriad of sleep problems caused by the pump running at night. This changed the way Yoav practiced. Instead of reflexively placing an order for a procedure, he thought about how a particular intervention would affect the patient's overall quality of life. In other words, he went beyond the textbook to consider not just the problem but the patient as well. As he considered each medical situation he encountered on his rotation, he weighed not just risks and benefits but also implications and impact.

Making rounds, Yoav would ask questions related to quality of life, thinking more of the individual in front of him than how such a scenario would be presented in a textbook. Having a better understanding of the meaning of complications, he began to ask questions about the difference between managing an esophageal leak with a second operation and managing it by placing a stent. He would talk about what could go wrong with each procedure he suggested and how that might affect the patient. As a matter of fact, all of my residents started doing this after attending the support group. And what a difference it made to their understanding of both disease and longitudinal patient care.

Knowing the impact of having a leak and the ways in which having to manage that leak might disrupt daily life, my teams became more thoughtful, more creative, and more open about how we discussed cases and found solutions. This deeper understanding also started to connect my residents back to the "why" of what we do and how we change lives for the better. We were preventing burnout.

I learned from treating Doyle, aka the Marlboro Man, that looking toward the future with the aim of being proactive is what real surgeons do. When I was treating Doyle, I tried to take a 360-degree view of things, not just to understand what had gone wrong in the past but to get a sense of what was *likely* to go wrong in the future. Specifically, I considered all of the complications that can occur with a stent and tried to figure out how to fix his existing stent to prevent migration. Visions of the future and what might happen become clearer as we gain experience. Young, inexperienced surgeons have a difficult time imagining the consequences of their interventions with the same degree of clarity.

When we communicate all of the difficult things that might happen after surgery or because of surgery, we call this "laying crepe"—an old-fashioned term that describes how a mortician would begin laying crepe into the coffin to prepare for a body. Explaining these potential consequences to patients and family members helps ensure that they have a full understanding of the different pathways involved during a procedure. Providing them with this information helps them to make an informed decision as to whether to proceed with surgery, and to truly understand the potential consequences of that decision. This helps patients and families deal with those bad outcomes if they happen. The worst thing that can happen is to have a bad outcome no one anticipated. If the first time they are hearing about a complication is when it is happening, patients and their families are alarmed and have had no time to prepare.

Seasoned surgeons also understand the importance of anticipating those complications and doing things to prevent them from happening. A good example would be placing a feeding tube when you anticipate that the patient might have a difficult recovery. For example, if the patient does develop a leak, they become sick and septic, and often are too ill to have a feeding tube placed. That means they have to have a tube placed through their nose and throat into their stomach for feeding. The placement of that tube through such a long passage is uncomfortable, and it could also erode into adjacent structures, leading to more complications. If the patient simply had a feeding tube placed in the beginning, in anticipation of a potential leak, circumstances might not become dire. Making sure patients have good nutritional status, undergo any necessary rehabilitation to make them stronger before surgery, and are given a blood thinner to prevent a blood clot are ways that we can prevent catastrophic complications at the time of surgery. Being proactive and coming up with a preventative strategy is always better than playing a reactive catch-up game.

Personally, I'm concerned not just with safety but also with efficacy. You can turn every potential patient away from surgery and be considered a "safe" surgeon because you won't have any bad outcomes. We call this "cherry picking." If you want to be a good surgeon and make a difference in the world, you have to take risks. You have to weigh the consequences of your intervention against the risk of not operating. You have to know your boundaries and—this is important—you have to know if someone else might be able to do something better.

Weighing what you offer against what other specialties might offer is important. For example, some drugs might have a better outcome than your surgery. It's up to you to know that—and to keep knowing that. When I am looking to add someone to my team, I look for surgeons who are forward-looking, who anticipate complications and proactively take measures to prevent those complications from happening in the first place. I look for surgeons who understand competitive technology and know when to turn a patient over to a technology that might serve that patient better than surgery, even when it might mean they lose revenue, RVUs (relative value units, which are used to support the calculation of physician time, workload, practice expense, and liability protection), or caseload. Surgeons are far more than a simple RVU.

Furthermore, I look for providers who are also setting themselves up for success in the event that a complication occurs. Because it will. For example, it's important to spare the latissimus and serratus muscles when you do a thoracotomy so that if a patient does end up with a leak you have abundant muscle to patch that leak with. Not all surgeons understand how important it is to preserve those muscles for later use, which is why so many patients suffer by having to undergo a further procedure to solve an additional complication that need not have happened in the first place. Some surgeons fail to learn the modern techniques to navigate safely through a surgery with a minimally invasive approach and instead create giant incisions, cutting the chest wall muscles in half and leaving the patient with a higher chance of developing post-thoracotomy pain syndrome.

Yoav got to see that firsthand. And that made him a better surgeon. He was both excited and energized to learn about the more personalized side of survivorship. His line of questioning, excitement about cases, and questions about deciding which surgery to perform changed and intensified from that point on. Interestingly, I think as a result of this support group, in combination with the great experiences we provided, almost every year a general surgery resident chose to enter into a career to specialize in cardiothoracic surgery when I was at Houston Methodist Hospital.

Being a part of our surgery team and participating in the support group didn't just teach our residents about surgery. What they learned from our longitudinal patient group inspired them. I have stayed in touch with almost all of my residents throughout the years. When I asked them what inspired them to go into the specialty after doing a rotation with us on general surgery, they frequently mention the support group, the teamwork, and the experience overall. They found it so inspirational, they felt like they wanted to do that for the rest of their life, no matter how hard it would be.

Nine

A Union of Forces

A complex esophageal reconstruction, which typically lasts six to twelve hours, unites four professions and deploys an assortment of precision equipment, like a special forces unit on a mission. Each player has a role and a goal. Each has their own equipment and specialty, yet they must work together as a single entity or lives will be lost. A mistake by one team member could mean the death of a patient.

The thoracic surgeon starts in the abdomen by dissecting the bowel and laying out the blood supply to make sure the roots of the vessels are good enough for rearrangement. She may also have to work in the chest to prepare room for the connection of the esophagus to the new conduit (made of small intestine, colon, or stomach tissue) that will carry food to the abdomen. She will often remove part of the chest wall, ribs, and tissue to make room for the patient to swallow. The microvascular plastic surgeon may have to take vessels from the chest, typically used for heart bypass, and instead prepare them for bowel bypass to keep the new organ—now functioning as an esophagus—alive. Often this part happens with both surgeons working across the table from each other in sync. Reimplanting the blood supply is done under an operating microscope by a microvascular plastic surgeon. Gastroenterology teams may have to perform an endoscopy to make sure the remaining esophagus is healthy. Hepatobiliary teams (those who focus on surgery of the liver, pancreas, and bile duct) may be needed, and sometimes, when the lower part of the GI tract has to be utilized, a colorectal surgeon will be called in. Through all of this, the anesthesiologist orchestrates a balance between sedation, ventilation, maintenance of oxygenation, and perfusion to the body with good blood pressure, often following customized pathways that are built on evidence and experience.

Because rebuilding the esophagus when a traditional stomach tube is not an option is so difficult to perform, only a few places in the world can perform this operation. At Mayo Clinic, we can do two in a day. Teams run between rooms, exchange duties, drop in when needed, and exit as others take over. We've done so many of these surgeries that we have perfected the sequence of a typical complex reconstruction. Pathways and checklists define our sequence of events, algorithms define the management of anesthetic, and time-tested protocols enable these cases to feel almost routine. Almost.

What looks to the patient to be a bespoke, complex, unique event—something they regularly call a "miracle"—is really the manifestation of practice, scientific discovery, trial and error, root cause analysis, and hours upon hours of supportive teamwork. (I actually like to call this phenomenon a "scientarvel." A totally made-up word, it speaks to the science of the miracles/marvels that regularly happen at Mayo.) Being a part of an experienced unit that works together to enable extraordinary outcomes is one of the highlights of a surgeon's career—if she is fortunate enough to experience it.

When a team comes together in the operating room, talk often becomes unnecessary. Communication can occur with just a nod. An experienced scrub nurse will place what you need into your hand because they've seen you work a thousand times and know exactly what is required and when. They might even know what you need better than you do. My scrub nurse, Jaymie, knows every step of my cases as well as I do, if not better. The circulating nurses, like Keri, know how to stock the room and grab equipment you might not even anticipate using, but they do.

When we are all working at our best, these steps happen in the correct order and turnover is quick. We have briefings that enable healthy discussion and complete preparation, in addition to something we like to call "time-outs," in which we draw attention to any areas where a mistake might be made. At the end, we do a debriefing to review what went well and what went wrong. Then we make a plan to do better next time.

Competent teams often might not even consciously be aware of all the tasks they are completing. It's like a symphony. Time melts away and a case seems to take a few minutes, when in reality it might be hours. Often you are concentrating so hard that you won't feel hunger, won't feel the need to use the bathroom, or won't even know when you are going into labor—all of which have happened to me. Mihaly Csikszentmihalyi describes this phenomenon in his book *Flow* as "that optimal experience when people experience deep enjoyment, creativity, and a total involvement with life."[1] During "flow," a functional MRI will show the "joy" parts of your brain (right frontal cortex, precuneus, left amygdala, and the left insula) lighting up like a Christmas tree. He pointed to surgeons as one of those groups most likely to experience the sense of flow.

But not all teams are created equal or run the same way. Having operated in multiple hospitals throughout my career, I have had the opportunity to see when a surgeon's time is used wisely—and when it is not. A surgeon should be operating all day, but long OR turnover times, case bumping, poor schedule optimization, and lack of attention to detail put valuable teams on hold and place surgeons on the bench, to say nothing of the deleterious effects this has on patients.

All of us want to feel optimized, to give the best we can for as long as we can. It's hard to experience peak effectiveness when we are not engaging at full capacity, when long wait times and constant interruptions are chipping away at productivity and creating frustration. These frustrations mount and make people feel that their skills—and their time—are not valued. Not working with a dedicated team can be a big frustration and an impediment to productivity. When I operated in Houston I worked with many different teams. This meant that I had to consciously negotiate how to conduct each case and orient new members each time someone appeared in the room for the first time. There was a lot of explanation and a lot of repetition. That can wear on a surgeon.

Arriving at Mayo Clinic, I learned that I would be working with the same main team almost every operating day, with the exception of the occasional staff member who would call in sick or take vacation. The team was first-rate, and at first it seemed perfect. But then I realized that a few of the members could have been better selected for the type of surgery I performed. For instance, the professional assistant I was assigned initially was more interested in helping with open surgery than with robotic and minimally invasive techniques.

It's hard to overestimate the value of a good professional assistant. They're the people who bring a patient into the OR and help position them on the operating table to ensure that arms and legs don't get injured after hours of being in the same position. Not only do they assist with getting the equipment in the room ready, but they will also assist in the operation itself, sometimes holding the camera for minimally invasive surgery and at other times holding big retractors. A professional assistant will free up the nurse to get medications and circulate around the room and just generally have the surgeon's back. I should know. My current professional assistant, Cassie, is a godsend. My eyes and ears, the protector of my patients, she will change the camera angle without me even asking to give me a better view. She reminds me to do countless things every day. And not just me. She will, for example, make sure the anesthesiologist pulls the nasogastric tube back before I staple the stomach to make the conduit, preventing me from accidentally stapling across the tube. As I said, a godsend.

When I arrived at Mayo, I was grateful that a seasoned professional assistant was assigned to my team. Yet as much as he gave me his all, we both knew that my specialty wasn't his first choice. So when I learned that one of my partners who predominantly did open surgery was looking for a new assistant, we came up with a transfer deal that allowed me to recruit someone who was more interested in what I was doing. It worked out better for everyone.

There will always be adjustments wherever humans are involved. But over time I found that working with a dedicated unit enabled me to develop a deep understanding of how my team worked. The group of people I worked with was stable and dedicated both to the process and to the patient, which allowed me to become attuned to them and align with their technical skills and their communication styles. We never took anything for granted, but there was a sense of predictability that made everything go that much more smoothly.

Working consistently with the same people enhances efficiency. Numerous studies have shown how dedicated operating teams are "associated with improvements in mortality, turnover time, teamwork, communication and costs."[2] My experience bears that out. I once went back and looked across the span of a year at a single type of case, comparing productivity, turnover time, and operating time within that specific case type. I found that by working with a dedicated team we were able to complete surgery an average of forty-five minutes earlier than with a secondary or ad hoc team, no matter how good those teams were. We never published this data, although it proved to be statistically significant. But we acknowledge the value of dedicated teams and the role they play in making miracles happen.

If there's one thing I've learned from my experience building teams throughout my career, it's that communication is the cornerstone of teamwork. Not to mention having a shared focus and a common set of goals. At Mayo our mission is "to inspire hope and contribute to health and well-being by providing the best care to every patient through integrated clinical practice, education and research." That's a lofty intention, and you'd be hard-pressed to find someone who disagrees with it. But it doesn't sound all that different from most other hospital mission statements. I'm more of a fan of an earlier statement by William Mayo, who in 1910 said, "The best interest of the patient is the only interest to be considered, and in order that the sick may have the benefit of advancing knowledge, union of forces is necessary."

Sometimes that union works seamlessly. Not always. I would be lying if I said I was never discriminated against, bullied. sexually harassed, hit on the head with a medical chart (yes, really), or overworked and undersupported. It all seemed to be a part of the journey, but it shouldn't be. We need to do better at protecting people, especially those who are not in positions of power. We need to have systems in place that safeguard everyone. But it's not always a systems issue. We are human, and that means we are falli-ble. I know there are things I have done that have left others feeling alienated or disrespected, feeling as if I didn't value them or their contribution. I may have spoken brusquely or expected more from someone than they were able to give. I may have ignored someone I should have acknowledged, and I may have assumed . . . well, too many things. This has never been my intention, but sometimes our intentions and actions get tangled, especially in moments of high drama, which the hospital is full of.

I expect a lot of myself and need a lot from my team. Sometimes I am bad at setting boundaries, perhaps because selectively dropping some of these boundaries has given me insight and allowed me to know my patients on a deeper level. This has enabled me to feel more connected and has helped me to have an even better under-standing of how my patients struggle. I am grateful that my family understands that I cannot just flip a switch and cut myself off from patients when I get home. For example, I give all of my patients my cell phone number. I know I am not supposed to do that, but they respect my time and only reach out personally to me when they fall through the cracks. Falling through these cracks after such a serious surgery can be life-threatening. I want to be that safety net and be there for them. However, this can create a swirl of stress for team members who support me. Because I give so much of myself and expect so much from my teams, the job can be overwhelming for many. Sometimes I am not aware of the toll it takes on those around me. I tend to forget not everyone is leaning in to the same degree.

When I know I have acted poorly, I apologize and do what I can to remedy my error. I try to own up to what I have done. People can be tough to understand. When someone has acted unkindly or unprofessionally toward me, I try to place myself in their position, to imagine what could possibly have happened to them to make them act so unreasonably. What was it that made them think that their unacceptable behavior was acceptable? I try to imagine how much they must hurt inside and hope that my compassion for them can be greater than the frustration that might arise whenever they act out. This is how we support one another. We forgive, stand up for, defend, and advocate for each other. And we make it clear that certain behaviors will not be tolerated. Especially when a life is at stake.

Long before I learned about the importance of boundaries, I found out that I was going to be working with a legendary surgeon I had always looked up to. A supporter of younger practitioners and a leader within his own institution, he was a giant in national society leadership as well. He seemed approachable and unassuming, despite holding tremendous power.

"You're going to love working with him, Shanda," one of my colleagues told me. "He's a terrific man and you'll learn a lot."

Yes, as it turns out, I did learn a lot. But not what I had expected. Our relationship started out strong. We were in the same workgroup and collaborated on a few projects. He assigned me tasks that I happily took on, including writing papers and representing our group at conferences. When he asked me to take the lead on one particular project, I was elated. I felt like he saw potential in me and trusted me to do a good job.

I was thrilled by the interest this celebrated leader showed in my career. But as I started to grow as a surgeon, coming into my own, I noticed a shift in our relationship. When I spoke up in larger groups, I could tell by his body language that he didn't approve. This normally welcoming man could adopt a stern demeanor that tele-graphed his displeasure. He would actually bristle when I advocated for a project I was passionate about or tried to initiate something without obtaining his approval before the meeting. God forbid I talk about the particular challenges facing women in surgery.

His dissatisfaction wasn't limited to the meeting room. More than once this leader called me after a meeting had ended to tell me he didn't like the way I brought things up. "I don't think you handled that well," he would say, adding, "You're young. You'll learn." He felt like I challenged him, that I was too vocal in my disagree-ment. I wanted to attend society meetings to get a better view of my profession, to understand the perspective of my colleagues, *all* my colleagues. My mentor wanted unwavering support and acted as if any question or contradiction was a betrayal. I wanted to learn to find a way to advocate effectively and bring others along with me, but I didn't want to make enemies along the way. It was a fine line I would need to learn to walk. Being a part of a group with strong-minded leaders means you have to learn to support them while at the same time not losing your voice.

The intimidation worked for a bit; I was reluctant to speak up. But, after sitting quietly for a few meetings, I realized that I had earned my right to be at the table. I had worked hard to enter my profession and become a leader within the national society. I cared about my colleagues and my patients. I gave them almost everything. How could I make a difference sitting there like a wallflower? Holding back on the questions I needed to ask or the suggestions I wanted to offer was doing nobody any good. Nor was it in my nature. Sitting quietly might have gained the favor of the executive council or the nominating committee and might have helped me move ahead, but it was not the right thing to do. I had to question myself and ask why I was there in the first place. I was there to make a difference, to bring in more diversity and make people feel more included.

I decided to be honest and respectful. I spoke my mind and tried to stand up for those who were not in the room, mostly the women who were struggling to find a place in cardiothoracic surgery. When I entered the field of cardiothoracic surgery in 2003, women accounted for less than 3 percent of our specialty. Today that number has doubled to 6 percent. But there are still too few of us at the mid- and senior-level rank sitting around the leadership table.

After being in the profession for a while, I noticed that men and women handled things differently, both in and out of the operating room. That was one of the main reasons I wanted to be active in our professional societies. When it came to the OR, we all proceeded with skill and professionalism. Gender was irrelevant most of the time. But in the conference room, that all changed. Men tended to take up more time and space at our meetings. They interrupted more and talked over other participants. I knew that men were perceived as more logical and analytic than women—"intuitive" is a word often used to describe women—and that men are seen as more confident too. So I set about modifying the way I acted at our group meetings. I'd always been evidence-based in the issues I brought up, but I did more homework and tried to see things from a perspective that wasn't my own. I didn't bring up concerns lightly either. I researched the facts surrounding important initiatives so that I could offer more information and less opinion. And I was strategic, often asking guiding questions and allowing others to come up with solutions so that there might be more buy-in. It worked—most of the time. I didn't win every battle, but I felt heard, and I was getting a good response from my peers.

But this senior leader was in a category all his own. The man who had previously declared that he wanted to help me in my ca-reer continued to tell me to stop talking so much. Specifically, he resisted my attempts to broaden the leadership of the organization. I wasn't the only one who wanted to be represented by a more diverse group. With the exception of only one African American president, ours had been a mostly all-white male leadership—the only woman to gain the presidency was a posthumous appointment after she tragically died from pancreatic cancer. She would have been the first female president of the organization that governed the group of seven thousand cardiothoracic surgeons. This was the organization that purported to represent almost everyone within our specialty, but that representation was lacking diversity, and many of us were trying to address that.

Many of us, but not all.

This senior male leader called me out when, after observing that a lot of committees featured the same familiar faces, I suggested a one-person/one-appointment policy. I was disappointed that he couldn't see how a more inclusive membership would only help to advance the specialty. (I now belong to and help govern a working group that focuses on diversity, equity, and inclusion in our specialty.) Still, I continued to push for diversity, and I continued to advocate for women. I wanted to continue to create scholarships to encourage more women to become involved in our specialty. I pressed for things like breastfeeding stations for the female surgeons who attended our sessions or the ability to present at meetings via Skype or Zoom when in the postpartum phase.

The need for this occurred to me as I was walking through the halls at our annual meeting and discovered one of my female colleagues balancing a cumbersome backpack as well as her purse and laptop bag. With everything she was burdened with, this young surgeon looked more like a pack mule than the medical professional she was. I stopped to chat with her, at which point she told me that she was getting ready to give a talk but needed to pump—hence the large backpack with all of her pumping equipment. It's like that observation about Ginger Rogers doing everything Fred Astaire did, but backward and in heels. The poor woman was juggling it all and not complaining a bit—taking it all in stride and doing her best to get through the hardships, much like the rest of us did.

Giving a talk to fellow cardiothoracic surgeons is stressful enough; add breastfeeding, being separated from your child, and hormonal changes on top of that . . . well, that would elevate anyone's stress level. I tried to support this colleague—and others like her—by bringing up the issue in the board meeting. Luckily, despite the attitude of a few members, the motion received overall support and at the next national meeting, we had breastfeeding stations. I know that doesn't seem as radical as it was at the time, with breastfeeding pods now located at every major institution, but when we discussed it and decided to offer designated areas for such activity, it was somewhat radical.

Finally, we were making progress. With breastfeeding stations at every meeting, scholarships, grants, novel initiatives, and more women on the board, we were making real changes. I thought we had turned a corner. Not that we didn't have a long way to go. As I became more experienced and comfortable with these leaders, I hesitated less to bring up these issues. After ten-plus years as a surgeon, I could see how things were changing, how some of the stodgier members of our group were coming around to a new way of thinking. Then I received a phone call from my male leader colleague.

"Shanda," he said, "you have got to stop with these female issues." He was angry now, unleashing his temper on me. "People are . . . well, how should I put it. People are sick of hearing about it."

"Excuse me?" I couldn't believe what I was hearing.

"This is overshadowing your career. Why can't you be more like"—and here he mentioned a senior female colleague who was nearing retirement. I had a great deal of respect for that doctor. She came of age at a different time and with an entirely different set of circumstances. I shudder to think of what she had to put up with as she paved the way for so many young women to follow her. But that doctor, in spite of her incredible achievements in the field, never became a leader within our major specialty societies, and especially was never a leader within the group that this male colleague represented. Like many women of her generation, she never had to contend with the push and pull of family and career because she felt she had to sacrifice one for the other. She didn't have the choices I had, choices that—I was well aware—came about in no small part due to the efforts of women like her.

I was grateful to my predecessor, but I didn't want to emulate her. I had the right to conduct my career in the way that I thought best, to speak about the issues that mattered to me and the other members of my profession. I did my best to defend myself as my former mentor told me that I could make a more impactful change if I just "kept my head down and continued to do the work." He told me women should just stand out with their scientific accomplishments rather than trying to implement change or call out inequity.

It was sexism, pure and simple. You can be a female surgeon as long as you don't draw attention to being female, to being *different*. It was up to me to fit into the existing structure, a structure built for and by men. It reminded me of the time when, as a general surgery resident, I asked to have smaller sterile gloves on the nursing stations to grab for bedside procedures. Before I came, the stock was limited to size eight—typically worn by men. When I put the large gloves on my hands I looked like Minnie Mouse. This added a whole level of difficulty to the placement of a central line or any other bedside procedure. When I made the request, I was told to carry my own gloves around in my pocket so I would have what I needed. I wasn't asking for anything out of the ordinary. I simply wanted gloves that fit. Apparently that was too much to ask for. The calls telling me to "stop with the female issues" reminded me of that incident, one that took years to resolve. (Not until one of my program directors took on the issue were smaller sterile gloves routinely stocked on the floor.)

I told no one about what this senior surgeon said to me, but inside, I started to wonder if I was approaching things in the right way. This illustrious surgeon made me question my approach and, frankly, almost everything I had done. He seemed to be warning me that if I continued down the path I was traveling, I would be asked to leave my role in society leadership after my term ended. The issues I brought up were irritating, I presumed. I started to doubt myself and to question my effectiveness—for a while.

I had put in so much work and time. I had poured my soul into helping this group. Was I no longer fit to lead because I was too passionate about inclusion of women? Had I pushed too hard?

How did they see me? I knew that I would rather err on the side of passion than submission any day.

Then I got angry. How dare he speak to me like that? How dare he question my intentions? If this leader wouldn't support my efforts, then it was up to me to advocate for myself and for others. I had that right. (Today, I understand the gift of feedback and perspective, diversity of thought, and the value of bringing more women into our specialty. Our unique perspective enhances the specialty and is a rising tide that raises all boats.)

Over time it became clear to me what was happening. My advisor was part of the old guard and had benefited from a hierarchical structure that was being dismantled. The medical profession was changing rapidly, and perhaps he saw me as a threat. When there were two levels of rank between us and I was at the beginning of my career, a subordinate who could learn from him and look up to him, I was an ally. An acolyte, even. While he wanted to encourage my technical and research skills, he didn't necessarily want to see me as an equal. That was a level of the pyramid reserved for a select few.

Ten

A Second Opinion

When patients come in for a second opinion for any disease, they're often looking to escape a burning house. Everyone wants the highest-quality healthcare and the most advantageous results. Often patients go from surgeon to surgeon with little to no comparative information to allow them to make the best choice for their surgery. Of course, "best" is a relative term and depends on so many quality measurements—not just who has the most experience or the highest ranking but who has the best hospital support system to intervene in the event things go wrong.

Not every patient seeks further help, though. Some people may feel defeated by their diagnosis and by the prospect of what's ahead. Others may see a way forward but lack the ability or resources to get there. Or they don't want to insult the doctor or surgeon they've already seen and feel they have no other option than to take what is given. Others rely on their primary care providers or referrals from caregivers who may not understand the intricacies of their situation. Instead of looking for the best surgeon for them, some patients might be struggling to find one at all. And while it may be true that research is helpful to many people, for some it can be overwhelming and may end up delaying their decision. Then there are the patients who lack the wisdom or skill to do that kind of research and blindly trust for the sake of convenience or through magical thinking.

Approximately five thousand esophagectomies are performed in the United States every year. That number should be higher. Much higher. Unfortunately, too few patients are referred for the surgery, even when they are strong candidates. Sometimes this is because they cannot travel to a healthcare center that can perform the surgery, other times they do not have access to sophisticated groups who recognize the benefit and role that surgery plays. Fewer still realize that they are three times more likely to survive the surgery if they go to centers that do a large number of these surgeries than if they go to a small-volume program that might be closer to home and seemingly more convenient. Allowing a generalist to perform a highly specialized and difficult surgery is frequently not in a patient's best interest. Unfortunately, it often seems like patients would need their own medical degree in order to have all the information they need to make the best decision. Patients fall victim to marketing schemes that advertise things like "robotic surgery" or "close to home," each of which often has nothing to do with the quality of surgery or the ultimate outcome. A surgeon can do just as much harm to a patient using a robot as with their own hands. I have seen it.

We also need to differentiate among three things: patient assessment of surgeons and hospitals, rankings, and outcomes from surgery. Patient-reported experience measures (PREMs) capture the patient view of what happened during the healthcare visit or hospitalization and is an assessment that evaluates and monitors service delivery. Patient-reported outcome measures (PROMs) capture the impact of an illness or health condition from the patient perspective, without interpretation or interference from a provider. PROMs are used to monitor the health condition over time and the effectiveness of treatments and interventions. Together, PREMs and PROMs measure the scope of a patient's experience from the time of hospitalization to the end of their illness. All of these things need to be more transparent, and patients need better access to high-quality information in a language they can understand, presented to them in a way that makes sense.

People often conduct research by asking others for their opinions or recommendations. And there are many outlets to assist, such as the ranking systems from *US News and World Report*, the Society of Thoracic Surgeons quality outcomes database, and the American College of Surgeons (ACS) National Surgical Quality Improvement Program (NSQIP), to name a few. Each of these systems purports to measure the quality of a hospital or program to assist patients in selecting the best choice for their healthcare. But the best choice isn't available to all. Not everyone can afford a plane ticket, rental car, and hotel to travel to the number one hospital in the nation. Those with less are filtered out. Not everyone has insurance, and many can't afford the most basic healthcare. There is a wide disparity in our country between those who have resources and those who do not, and it can be hard to find the most appropriate care. I won't even begin to talk about the disparity between countries, comparing our own country and our resources with those of underdeveloped nations, where even basic needs like water and food are a problem and healthcare takes a backseat.

Many people don't know how to advocate for themselves. They find the medical profession intimidating and shut down when they get in the doctor's office That wasn't the case with my patient Jack. He was an engineer, and as I've learned over the years, engineers are easy to pick out of a crowd. They typically arrive early to the clinic with a typed list of their problems, have read every article on the topic of their disease, and take meticulous notes. Presenting their surgeons with an alphabetized index of the physicians and specialists they've consulted, engineers will tell you what they ate the day before with precision and accuracy, as if detailing a structural analysis. They are great at following directions.

Jack was like this. An aerospace engineer at NASA, he was referred to me because he was seeking someone who had a reputation for being passionate about esophageal cancer. He said that when he asked around, my name came up in several circles. Jack grilled me at our first meeting. There's no other way to put it. He wanted to know how many cases I had done, how often I misjudged things, and how I evaluated my skills. Was I better than others? In what areas? I appreciated the questions. It meant he had done his homework and knew how to find a good surgeon. He was meticulous. I always appreciate when patients are smart enough to go for a second opinion or when they know to seek answers to good and relevant questions. This lets me know they are invested and more likely to make the effort to recover as well.

It turns out Jack had scheduled a colonoscopy after an examination with his physician, an exam in which he shared that he had experienced some reflux in the past. His physician told him that since he was going to have the sedation and the colonoscopy, perhaps they should scope his esophagus as well, just to be on the safe side. Jack agreed, and the incidental finding saved his life. He'd had just a little bit of reflux, no trouble swallowing, and no weight loss. Too many patients are diagnosed late in their disease and do not present for endoscopy to diagnose esophageal cancer early enough. Too few patients know that years of reflux can lead to progression to cancer.

Jack seemed lucky, and the cancer appeared to be what we call T1a—the earliest form of invasive cancer. This stage of cancer is in the innermost part of the lining of the esophageal lumen. It has yet to invade the muscular part of the wall. Typically, we would just go in with endoscopy and scoop out the cancer from the inside, after which we would look for any remaining cancer characteristics in the lymph nodes and the surrounding tissue. That is the exact procedure that would be offered if Jack came into any hospital today. For staging the cancer—that is, determining what stage the cancer is at—we'd use different imaging studies, like ultrasound, CT (computed tomography) scans, and PET (positron emission tomography) scanning. The ultrasound uses sound waves to give us a good look at the structures inside the body. The CT scan combines a series of X-rays taken from different angles to scan the entire chest, neck, abdomen, and even pelvis. The PET scan measures sugar uptake in rapidly dividing cells to identify infections or cancer. Most patients who pass through this gauntlet of scans and show no evidence of advanced disease feel confident enough to believe their cancer is limited and an endoluminal procedure should be safe.

Not Jack. We had talked about doing an endoscopic ultrasound (EUS), using a probe that we would pass down into the esophagus to look at lymph nodes beyond the esophagus walls. Although it's not a perfect technique, this can show us much more than what we can see with merely a camera inside the lining of the esophagus. Jack persisted because he wanted to have all the details to make the best decisions, and he knew how important staging was. I am pretty sure he had already looked up the American Joint Committee on Cancer staging handbook as well as the National Comprehensive Cancer Network guidelines. We discussed surgery too.

Jack was not a risk taker. He wanted to know how accurate the EUS was. He specifically asked me how many times I had seen it be wrong. He wanted to do everything he could to uncover even the smallest evidence of disease, and that meant leaving no stone unturned. It was like he was planning on launching a rocket and wanted nothing left to chance.

The staging of esophageal cancer is notoriously inaccurate. Even though we can use things like CT scan, PET scan, EUS, and endoscopy, 30 percent of the time or more we are wrong, especially when the tumor looks like it is going into the muscular layer of the esophagus wall (what we call T2). Determining whether or not cancer is involved in lymph nodes is even more unpredictable. We can pick out malignant lymph nodes that are large or have enough tumor in them to make the PET scan light up, but I suspect that we miss a lot of cases where the lymph nodes have smaller amounts of disease, and thus we often underestimate the degree of disease. For instance, a PET scan can detect cancer within a lymph node only if the tumor is at least 8 mm in size.

My patient did the math. Even if there was a less than 10 percent chance of undetected cancer in the lymph nodes, it was a chance he was not willing to take. No way was Jack going to play the odds. He calculated what might kill him and planned to carefully take out each possible risk factor. That meant surgery—he wanted an esophagectomy. He knew that if we went in and did an extensive lymph node dissection (which was part of the removal of the cancer and staging), we would have a better idea of whether or not cancer was involved in the lymph nodes. Jack knew that if there was cancer in those lymph nodes that went undetected, he would miss an opportunity to get chemotherapy or, at the very least, to be put more carefully under surveillance. He wanted all of the details and he was not willing to gamble with his life.

Well, our engineer turned out to be smarter than we all realized, because he had an undetected cancerous lymph node next to the celiac artery in his abdomen. Jack had presented to us with the type of cancer that rarely requires surgery, the type of cancer that would usually trigger a referral to a gastroenterologist to be scooped out from the inside. But without removal of the node, leading to a proper diagnosis and the possibility of receiving adjuvant treatment with chemotherapy after surgery, he might well have slipped through the cracks. Every gastroenterologist who scoops out a T1a cancer should tell their patient they have a 5-7 percent chance of having esophageal cancer that has already spread to the lymph nodes, cancer that can only be removed with surgery. Jack is alive today because he persisted to get the therapy he wanted.

Surgery is always a risk, but Jack took it because he knew it offered him the best possible chance of a cure. He had a radical attention to detail and knew what he wanted. It worked out well for him. He got as much of a guarantee of a cure as we can offer. He is alive today because of it.

Surgeons who perform only a few esophagectomies a year might want to consider not doing them. I don't do a few cardiac bypasses a year; if I did that, my complication rate would be impossibly high. Even though I am board-certified to do so, I don't do them at all, because I believe heart bypass surgery should be centralized and left to the experienced and actively practicing experts. Likewise with esophagectomy patients. That's the only way they will receive safer and more complete care. Let's face it: the complications are grave and the consequences are real.

So many of the patients I see with esophageal cancer get bad counseling. They go through diagnosis and staging, receive chemo-therapy and radiation therapy, then get restaged, and their doctors tell them it looks like the cancer is all gone. Although they might have started down the path of having chemoradiation with planned esophagectomy, they are sometimes guided away from the surgery. The statement that all the cancer is gone will be wrong more than half the time, and the patient may still have cancer—they just don't know it. Or they may be told they are not a good candidate for surgery, so they don't even take the next step to find out for sure whether this is true. They never go to see a surgeon and never consider surgery as an option.

Patients tell me repeatedly that their providers have told them not to opt for surgery. Perhaps their oncologists saw a bad outcome from an esophagectomy and want to spare them the pain. Perhaps providers just don't understand that 50 percent of the time when it looks like the cancer is gone, it is still lurking, waiting to come back with a vengeance. I hate meeting patients who were told they were cured only to find the cancer back and larger months after initial treatment. It makes my job harder and raises the risk of complications for those who can still undergo an operation. This is another reason additional perspective from a support group can help. You hear all of the stories and build a collective knowledge base. You are wiser because you can learn from the group.

I'm a surgeon. It's what I've dedicated my life to. And I love to operate. But I don't try to talk my patients into or out of surgery. After all, this is not about me. My job is to serve the patient. I do my very best to ensure that the people who come to me are educated and informed as to what is involved so that they can make the best decision *for themselves.* I let patients know that they always have a choice of treatment plan. And I'm proud to work for an organization that allows that to happen. At Mayo, all staff are salaried. We don't get paid per surgery, so there's no incentive to put people under the knife, as it were. We don't have to reach a quota or attain an RVU target, metrics that often are used when deciding on a surgeon's compensation. Tying compensation to RVU targets or quotas means that surgeons are motivated to perform surgery. Not at Mayo, where our salaried system supports our mission to provide the best evidence-based care to every patient. Taking away incentives for operative therapy over nonoperative therapy places the patient at the center of the conversation. That's as it should be.

I believe strongly that everyone should be given the opportunity to decide for themselves. I applaud patients who are willing to take a risk for a better chance of cure. I only wish we were better at delivering a balanced presentation to patients about their options. I wish that more doctors encouraged an open dialogue with their patients, allowing them the time to process the information they have received and the opportunity to come back later to discuss their options, after they have had a chance to do their own research—including a second opinion.

Most people come to me with their diagnosis already in hand. Because of this, I rarely have to share news of a diagnosis. However, I do sometimes have to tell patients about metastatic disease—disease that's too advanced for surgery to remove—or bad test results. I remember having to go into the room and tell one of our patients scheduled for an esophagectomy that he had metastatic disease and couldn't undergo the surgery. The news made him angry. "I did everything you asked," he said. "Everything. And it seemed like it was going so well." It was impossible for this patient to accept that there was metastasis, but it was there. His denial was natural. It's what people do as they slowly allow bad news to sink in. It is an essential stage of grief.

Giving a cancer diagnosis or news of worsening disease is awful. As I've mentioned, people seem to forget everything you say after they first hear the word "cancer," so I write everything on a white-board strategically placed in the patient's room or onto a piece of paper. I draw out the patient's journey and place little boxes next to each step so that we can track progress with a check mark. I write out all of the testing and the next steps, doing my best to show how we will make our decisions and what they might be. "If the rest of the staging tests demonstrate that you do not have metastatic disease, you will then likely start chemotherapy with radiation therapy. That might take about five weeks." Then it's another arrow from chemo-radiotherapy to "recovery," followed by another arrow leading to "surgery." After that I'll explain—with more boxes and arrows—what surveillance and survivorship might look like. At the bottom of the page, I tell them if they get to the point where the cancer does not come back at five years, they are finally pronounced cured. "That's when you plan a party. Because it certainly is worth celebrating." Because I am also an artist, I then draw a party hat.

My job is to take the patient from the top of the page to the bottom. I reassure them that I will be with them along their journey in some form or fashion. When I first meet with a patient, I spend a tremendous amount of time educating them on their diagnosis.

I also spend a lot of time explaining why it's a bad idea to go on the internet. The internet may provide a patient with information, but it also exposes them to advertisements from institutions whose aim it is to get them to change the course of their therapy or care. Unfortunately, many of these institutions can be predatory, attracting people at their most vulnerable moments. At Mayo Clinic, we aren't incentivized to keep patients within our institution or even to perform the surgery. We do not get a bonus for doing more operations, seeing more patients, or generating more surgical income. Our goal is to meet the patient's needs. Sometimes a patient who comes to me for a second opinion has a great surgeon and care system near them. If they have already seen a good surgeon close to home and are looking for reassurance, I give it to them. I think of us as a community. Sometimes a patient just needs to hear that we think it is okay to have their treatment near home (if they are close to a good center), or whether we are willing to work with their local providers to deliver a coordinated care experience. This is patient-centered care rather than institution-centered care. Unfortunately, so many institutions have yet to see the importance of that model and how it serves the patient's interest.

I support my patients by giving them a list of resources with timely and accurate information. Mayo goes a step further. In order to help control the narrative, it has devised a program called Mayo Clinic Connect,[1] an online community that helps patients get answers to their questions, as well as see issues that others have brought up. Mayo Connect helps broaden a patient's perspective and provides a helpful point of reference for those who aren't sure where to start or what to do, without having to wade through pages of data or pop-up ads. This is much like a carefully curated social media experience backed by experts.

Statistics can be daunting, and they only tell part of the story. We all know that information found online can lack proper context (which can be downright damaging) and can be of poor quality (which can be downright dangerous). Since most people don't understand statistics, they misinterpret the numbers. Take, for example, the five-year survival rates. If a patient sees a 15 percent survival rate over five years listed for esophageal cancer—which is one of the citations people can find on the internet—they quite naturally become distraught and depressed.

But patients are not statistics. They are not 15 percent alive at the end of five years. That's why we need to remember that statistics are not meant to give patients an accurate prediction of whether or not they will be alive at the end of their disease course. Data offers comparison points to determine what's better: a treatment versus a control. Furthermore, in our current era of immunotherapy and novel targeted therapies, we are seeing improvements in care every year. The data used to generate that general five-year survival rate is, by definition, old and out-of-date. If patients look at old data and generalized large databases, they are not seeing the real picture.

Sure, averages may help us compare treatment options, but they're not that helpful for our patients. In fact, averages often confuse people. If a patient has a good chance of dying in the year to come, they need to know that information so they can make plans accordingly. If a patient has a driver mutation, meaning changes in the DNA sequence that cause cells to become cancer cells, they need to know that too. (Checking tumor tissue for driver mutations can facilitate identification of more targeted treatment.) However, when a patient comes in with a particular stage of cancer, I am still not sure they need to know the historical probability of whether they will be alive five years from now. What can they do with that information? Besides, statistics do not account for the very wide range of differences concerning patient care.

Patients coming to Mayo Clinic who follow best-practice guidelines and have surgery performed by experts have a very different survival rate compared with those who get average care across the nation.

My team is starting to look beyond the statistics to assess the questions and comments made by patients over time. For example, wanting to connect with people whose survivorship had taken them past the ten-year mark, we spent time calling every survivor from the 2000–2010 period. Putting it bluntly, we wanted to know who was alive and who was dead. It was then I discovered that our cancer registry had lost track of most of the patients, and that there was no survivorship clinic or survivorship program in place to measure where they are in their lives or if they have been cured of their cancer.

The fact that we did not have a standardized system that followed patients and allowed institutions to individually query their survival made cancer survivorship reporting impossible. Outside of the National Cancer Database (NCDB) and other programs that use data from which all personally identifiable information has been removed, this capacity does not exist. Thus, patients are left to look at bad statistics, infrequently and inaccurately reported statistics, and statistics presented to them in a way that is almost impossible to understand. For example, many of our patients are surviving longer or in larger numbers than reported in the literature. It's very rare for a patient with stage IV esophageal cancer to survive more than five years, but it does happen, and when it does, the five-year survival rate for that individual is 100 percent.

I tell my patients to stay away from looking at survival curves. I tell them to avoid participating in groups without an expert moderator, so that they don't follow advice from someone with little experience or even dangerous and inaccurate advice. Instead, I steer them toward patient-driven support groups with experts present during the discussion to ensure that the information passed along is scientifically accurate information. I myself regularly attend such a group, in addition to making a concerted effort to guide patients on Facebook pages and making sure the information exchanged is reliable.

I've also spent an inordinate amount of time working with the health education specialist at Mayo Clinic to build patient education material. We write everything at an eighth-grade reading level to ensure accessibility and readability for the largest number of patients. We make sure the content is reviewed by experts across the enterprise, updating it frequently so that it remains relevant to current practice. Added to that is a two-hour video visit, in which nurses teach patients what to expect when they have an esophagectomy, and a ninety-minute patient education video we send to patients to help them demonstrate to their families and caregivers what to expect when their loved one undergoes an esophagectomy. This information is meant to supplement what they hear in the clinic and what they get from a video we created to educate patients about esophageal cancer as well as a class we designed to teach patients about esophagectomy (taught by health education nurse specialists). Repetition helps.

All of the educational material is considered complementary and is geared toward helping a patient understand in a comprehensive manner what they can expect. In it we repeatedly go over potential complications so that the initial consultation, which is frequently overwhelming, can be spent mostly on answering questions rather than trying to provide new patients with a waterfall of information. This educational material also allows patients to write their questions out and acquire the information at their own pace. By the time they return to see me at the completion of chemoradiation treatment, they have had ample opportunity to ingest all of the educational materials and come back with meaningful questions as they recover from that chemoradiotherapy and prepare for surgery. In that way, we providers have more time to answer questions. Once patients have the surgery, they will need a whole new set of instructions to guide them on how to eat, stay hydrated, and live their new life.

I try to be as creative as I can and make sure that we approach patients through as many different dimensions as possible. When they go to the internet, they may get conflicting information that confuses them instead of helping them to understand what lies ahead. Some patients are able to understand the differences between treatment regimens and come back with questions about why one may be better than the other, but many people just find themselves confused. I try to prevent that by curating their information experience. This is just a part of how we have maintained a three-star rating within the Society of Thoracic Surgeons National Database and a number one national ranking in gastrointestinal surgery (from *US News and World Report*).

Patients need to be empowered to ask questions—a lot of them. They need to make lists and advocate for themselves. And we care providers need to be empowered to provide better solutions for our patients and advocate for them beyond the walls of our individual institutions, specific organizations, or even countries. Until we are able to provide a global platform of enabling technology and solutions, disparity will continue.

Eleven

The Patient's Voice

These days, it's extremely rare to see a patient come to the clinic alone. Most people arrive with a spouse, child, partner, or trusted friend. Having someone with them—someone who is *there for them*—is of immeasurable value. Not only can these allies take notes and help decipher complex information, but also they can provide moral support and a strong shoulder. I encourage my patients to record our visits, FaceTime with their children during the clinic interaction if necessary, and bring as many people into the experience as possible. A crowded room may be temporarily distracting, but communication is the cornerstone of support.

Connecting, relating, understanding, and involving everyone in the big discussions and decisions is imperative. While some people are willing to go to great lengths to ensure their own survival, others are not. It's a deeply personal choice based on so many things. When patients get sick, the conversations they have with their loved ones are often their anchor as they make important decisions. I try to make a contract with my patients to ensure they are willing to do what it takes to survive surgery and at least thirty days after. Although only about 1 percent of our patients die within thirty days from esophagectomy, that single death can be devastating. So the patient, their family, and I make a verbal contract or agreement acknowledging that we are undertaking what may be a risky surgery and that all agree to do what is necessary to get through a reasonable recovery and give the patient a chance to survive. There are few things worse for a surgeon than making the effort to save a patient only to have the family withdraw care because the patient looks bad, is on a ventilator, or is undergoing complex treatment—to say nothing of what the poor patient must endure.

When families get exhausted from sitting at the bedside for weeks, their reactions may become visceral, with judgment giving way to instinct and emotion. Loved ones are terrible about getting rest for themselves. They may become so tired and overwhelmed—frightened too, of course—that they have trouble making decisions or even thinking straight. Unfortunately, this means that sometimes family will withdraw care even when the patient has a reasonable prognosis and is in the process of improving. They may simply become too exhausted or fatigued to see the light at the end of the tunnel.

My bias is always in favor of the patient. How could it not be? I remember with deep sadness the times when I performed surgery on a higher-risk patient, but the patient experienced a complication after surgery and the family decided to withdraw care. Complications happen all the time after surgery. Some patients develop blood clots that can even travel to the lungs and cause breathing problems. Others may develop a leak where we connect the new swallowing tube to the other parts of the gastrointestinal tract. Some patients might aspirate food and develop pneumonia. About a third of our patients have cardiac arrhythmias. The riskier the surgery and the more vulnerable the patient, the more likely the patient is to suffer a complication. But a complication doesn't have to mean a death sentence, which is why patients need to have these candid conversations with doctors and family members before surgery takes place. Knowing what people want in the event they have a terrible complication is an important element of support for both the patient and the physician. The patient needs to go into treatment with eyes wide open, understanding—as much as it is possible to understand—the pros and cons of each procedure. This information gives patients a sense of autonomy and makes them feel seen and respected. And there is no support without respect. Likewise, when it comes to physicians, they need to know that the investment they are making of their time and skill will also be respected, that the resources of the institution and the team will not be cast aside at the first bump in the road. We can't wait to have this conversation when a patient becomes critically ill. By then, it will be too late.

There are basic rules that each provider has to negotiate with her patients before anything takes place. First, we need to make sure we review a list of complications that might happen. Second, we need to discuss what kind of life a patient expects to have after the surgery. (Patients who undergo a pneumonectomy—removal of an entire lung on one side—will never run a marathon, for example.) And third, we need to explain to the patient what hospitalization will entail, as well as what to anticipate as they make plans to go home. This is all on top of explaining their surgery and care plan, as well as how to get ready for their operation.

Remember, we have about thirty minutes to do this on top of making a connection with the patient, performing a history and physical, explaining the disease, obtaining consent for surgery, entering data in the electronic health record, discussing the possibility of a blood transfusion, and planning the extent of the surgery, which we schedule on that visit. It's not easy to raise the subject of what to do in the event of a complication or a less-than-positive outcome, but it's my job.

To put everything in context, I try to tell patients what the chances are that they might suffer a particular complication. For example, about a third of patients might have an arrhythmia after an esophagectomy, and we have a protocol for managing that. It does not necessarily mean something went wrong, nor does it portend a worse outcome. However, slightly less than 10 percent of our patients might develop a leak, and that can have major consequences. Some patients want to talk about the learning curve for surgeons and how many cases or how much experience one may have; some want clarification about who will be doing the operation (me versus a resident) or to confirm where they will be going for follow-up care after surgery.

It's also important to differentiate between short-term and long-term goals. For example, a patient who does not want to be on a ventilator permanently may nevertheless require temporary use of a ventilator when recovering from surgery. This is an important distinction, and one that must be made. If a patient is undergoing risky surgery on an airway and might need an artificial lung to support their breathing, we talk about the possibility of an ECMO (extracorporeal membrane oxygenation) machine—what it is and what it will do. In this procedure, blood is pumped outside of the body to a heart-lung machine that removes carbon dioxide and sends oxygen-filled blood back to tissues in the body. Essentially, it's an artificial lung. The chances are rare that such a complex machine will be needed for an elective surgery, but if I suspect we might be considering it or might need it, I always take the time to prepare the patient for the possibility. Although these types of conversations seem cumbersome, complex, and intricate, they are important to have while the patient has the ability to say what she does and does not want. It's all about managing expectations.

We can best support our patients by letting them know what is involved during surgery and recovery, and by giving them a clear view of what kind of life they can expect to have after surgery. No patient undergoing an esophagectomy with reconstruction will ever function exactly as they did before surgery, when they had a working esophagus. It just won't happen. Which is why we need to be clear on everyone's expectations before a patient signs up for the procedure. Not everyone wants to go the distance, and that is their prerogative. It's not unusual for people to become so overwhelmed by the concept of surgery that they choose a less invasive procedure like radiation or palliative therapy. That's a good thing to know—that a patient has made an informed decision to avoid one procedure or surgery in favor of another.

Everyone is different. Some patients just don't want to have an incision and would rather go for serial radiation treatments instead of surgery. In those circumstances, we explain to the patient and their family that radiation may cause damage that might take decades to manifest. Ribs may break, or there may be other collateral damage (such as scar tissue to surrounding structures and even scar tissue damaging blood flow to the heart muscle in the long term) that may prevent future surgery from ever being a possibility. Again, it's all about communication.

Recovery from surgery is hard, but if a patient can persevere to get through the discomfort and, yes, pain, they are often in a much better place thirty days out from their operation. That month of recovery is very much like climbing a mountain, and I don't like to see patients quit when they are only halfway up the summit. A family needs to understand this before making the enormous decision to "pull the plug"—that is, withdraw care. Taking such an extreme step when a patient has a reasonable chance of a good recovery is a tragedy in my book. This is why I do my best to include the family in decision-making, to ensure they know what the patient wants.

Unfortunately, the situation can get really complicated when palliative care teams and critical care doctors get involved. It's imperative that these teams—who tend to come in much later in the process—be kept informed about pre-operative discussions and patient expectations. The discussion a patient has with a palliative care team is much different from the conversation the patient has with me. The goal of palliative care is to limit suffering and help patients understand the options available to them—discussions that do not center around prolonging life. Their emphasis is more on quality of life, whereas the emphasis of surgery is on quantity of life. I argue both should be part of how we measure surgical success. The critical care experts are focused primarily on getting a patient through an acute event and managing intensive use of life-supporting resources. These critical care teams travel in packs of around ten people at a time and subscribe to more of a groupthink mentality. They hardly ever get to see patients recover and come back to say thank you to their medical team. Thus, each team comes with a unique perspective. Sometimes this can create confusion and disharmony in a patient's care.

One of my partners from Houston, Dr. Bridget Fahy, was so interested in the intricate relationship between complex surgical decision-making and end-of-life issues like this that she went back to school and certified as a palliative care specialist as well. Her unique perspective and understanding of surgical issues made me see how complex it can get. Her candid and strategic approach to patients in their time of need offered our team a dimension others lacked.

I remember discussing end-of-life issues with a patient, Dr. Lee, who had a rare cardiac tumor (a pulmonary artery sarcoma). Dr. Lee, who was an NIH-funded professor, came to my office with his wife and neurologist son. The four of us talked about Dr. Lee's condition in great detail, discussing what we would do, as well as any possible aftereffects or complications. We talked about how when a tumor exists within the artery that goes to the lung, we have to take the entire lung on one side. We also talked about how this surgery is difficult to recover from, and how a patient might require extreme support just to live because of the massive redirection of blood flow. Together we discussed the nature of the surgery, and whether or not Dr. Lee wanted extreme measures, such as having a tracheostomy (moving the airway tube down to the neck and out of the mouth), a ventilator, or an ECMO machine.

Dr. Lee wanted surgery, which involved opening the entire chest. He consented to us removing an entire lung if necessary, rebuilding the artery going to the other lung, and a cardiopulmonary bypass if necessary. And if it became essential to utilize ECMO, Dr. Lee would agree to that too. I talked with his wife and son about recovery. It would be a long and arduous process. I told them that he would be in the hospital up to a month, and there would be more care needed after that. Recovery is like driving on a gravel road, I said, where you will hit a lot of bumps along the way. I did my best to prepare Dr. Lee, as I prepared all my patients, so that he was not alarmed when he hit those bumps. He needed to fasten his seatbelt.

My patient was clear he wanted everything done. His family was clear he wanted everything done. I was clear he wanted everything done. However, after surgery, in the middle of recovery, when his lungs failed and he required ECMO, Dr. Lee started saying something different. My patient felt like he couldn't breathe, and he was having hallucinations. Panic set in. There were days when he begged to die. His wife became so distraught and angry that she screamed at the nurses and staff for "torturing" her husband and not letting him die. Dr. Lee's son was trying to get through residency to support his young family, so he had the least amount of time to spend with his father, but he too asked us to withdraw care. He saw his father suffering and thought he should be allowed to make the decision to die if that was his wish. It was grueling to watch.

The crisis heightened when the nurses came together and begged us to withdraw care. The entire ICU team was distraught and at one point seemed close to caving in. Should they actually consider withdrawing care? I reminded the team that the patient had asked to stay the course. It was uncomfortable and, yes, frightening for us all, but I felt that there was a route to recovery.

This had happened before. It happens all the time.

That's why the most important voice is that of the patient *before* surgery, the lucid and deliberate voice in which the patient communicates what they want to their family and care team. That's why it's important that the family be present at these discussions and why they need to understand the patient's wishes in no uncertain terms. We don't record these conversations; I often wish we did. Nevertheless, I've never had a family deny that the dialogue took place, although sometimes they have been known to try to "re-negotiate" if there are dark days after surgery.

Though the son's neurology residency was demanding and exhausting, he finally got some time away from work to come visit his father. He also was able to go home and try to help his mom calm down. While staying at his parents' home, he discovered a large volume of tablets of Valium in the bathroom cabinet. When he asked his mother about it, she confessed to having seen his father frequently dip into the medication whenever he was not feeling well.

That was it!

My patient didn't really want to die. He was withdrawing from his chronic use of benzodiazepines before he was admitted to the hospital. Not only was his mind not clear, but his panic was coming from drug withdrawal. We gave him medication, put him in restraints, and reassured him constantly. We explained what was going on, and the nurses took great care of him, easing him through withdrawal in order to stabilize him. Gradually, his hallucinations went away, and his agitation dissipated. With the withdrawal from benzodiazepines safely behind him, Dr. Lee came around. He stopped asking the nurses to let him die, and eventually recovered.

It was a difficult time for all of us. I recall that at times the nurses thought I was being too pushy in insisting on my patient's treatment. But they hadn't been in the room when I had the pre-operative discussion with him. They weren't aware of how firm he'd been in his choice of care, how clear he'd been in making his decisions. In an ideal world, the contents of these discussions would be shared with everyone caring for the patient after surgery. Alas, we do not live in an ideal world, and sometimes, since we have so much to document, we do not do the best job documenting these conversations. My patient had a PhD and was an immunology researcher. He understood the risks and was willing to take them. He knew it would be a rocky road but was braced for impact. I was too. No way was I going to abandon his wishes once we were in the thick of it all. In this particular course, it was the right thing to do.

After Dr. Lee had fully recovered, he got back to work in his lab and eventually published a landmark paper in *Nature*. I posted it proudly in the ICU and sent it around in email form. This was a huge win for everyone—and a reminder to the teams that had been pushing me to withdraw care of why I resisted their urging. We made a difference with our patient. It doesn't always turn out that well, and walking that line can be difficult. But we did our best and we did what our patient wanted. No one can do more than that.

Twelve

A Circle of Trust

Trust is an essential part of any good working team. People need to have faith in their teammates and the system that surrounds them, and they need to know that their organization is grounded in trust at every level. How can our patients trust us if we don't trust each other? And how can we grow in our profession if we don't feel safe enough to own up to our mistakes and if we don't trust enough to have an open dialogue at every level?

I have lost only a few patients in the operating room, and each time it was a major event—not just in my career but in my life as well. When I operated on a trauma patient who had been stabbed in the chest and then experienced a lethal blood loss on the OR table, I sent a letter to the reams of people who had touched the victim, making sure to acknowledge the efforts of the whole team. I called out things everyone else did well and made a list of what I hoped to accomplish in the future to improve the outcome. I wanted the good people I worked with to know that no one was to blame for the loss of that patient. I wanted them to trust that they were valued and safe. Without such an environment, we will never have effective improvement in our systems or our process. Being vulnerable in front of our teams is not weakness; rather, it exhibits strength and binds us together. The thing is, you can be vulnerable only when you trust.

Trust in the operating room is essential to creating a psychologically safe environment in which team members feel they can rely on their partners. But you can't just be a partner in the OR. You have to be one outside the OR too. That means supporting your colleagues—in effect, being an ally. This isn't a touchy-feely thing. It's not about playing on the softball team or bringing in donuts (or having a team dinner in the backyard), as nice as those things are. It's about being there for the people you work with, about understanding what it is they need to thrive, and about supporting them in their efforts. Supportive co-workers foster a better workplace culture, one in which everyone feels free to express their ideas, further their professional goals, and pursue new strategies for improved outcomes. Supportive workplaces are more efficient. They run with minimal conflict, have stronger overall performance, and show higher levels of employee retention. Of course, there's always dissonance and disagreement, but it's how they're managed that's important. I have had the experience of seeing both good and bad leaders. Good leaders provide direction and inspiration and guidance. They demonstrate humility and commitment, and in so doing, they create safe workspaces. Bad leaders seem uncomfortable creating those safe workspaces. They don't speak up, advocate, or intervene when things go awry. They permit circuitous conversations, blame, punish, shame, and micromanage. They may not give you the support that you need. They may make you feel like you have a target on your head. Instead of inspiring you, you feel defensive or backed into a corner. They cannot see you the way you see yourself. The presence of such dissonance can degrade trust, suck the oxygen out of the room, and leave people in a tailspin. Some type of interruption must take place if a situation like that is going to be rescued.

Some groups are proactive enough to create codes of conduct to manage interactions and prevent things from spinning out of control. These directives go a long way toward creating supportive work environments. One of the best teams I have ever had the honor of working with is within the Center for Digital Health at Mayo Clinic, led by Dr. Brad Leibovich and Rita Khan, where, during a strategic retreat, we developed a draft of a manifesto to manage situations like these. This manifesto came from a situation in which someone was disrespectful of another person and no one said anything. Later, we applied the guidelines of the manifesto to the situation to get the people involved to start talking, and they all agreed the behavior was out of line. The person who was offended deserved better. She deserved to have an upstander say something, explore the situation with curiosity, and question the bad behavior. (In its simplest terms, an upstander is someone who acts in defense of a person who is the target of harm or injustice. Basically, it's someone who stands up for another, and the opposite of a bystander.)

Likewise, the person who offended had a right to understand what they did and to be called out, because feedback is a gift you give someone you care about. It would be equally tragic to keep the offender uninformed about the situation, allowing things to unravel.

This concept is at the heart of good leadership. Early intervention with timely, specific, behavioral feedback enables potential offenders to respond and change course. Nothing will upset the balance of a relationship more than going to someone months or years after something has happened with vague, nonspecific, inactionable negative feedback. It is as damaging and traumatic to the person delivering that type of feedback as it is to the one receiving it. I learned this in high school, in college, while working as a camp counselor, in premarital counseling with our pastor, and then in all of my leadership training throughout my career. Why do people struggle so much with this concept?

At the Center for Digital Health, we realized that some type of code was needed to enable people to feel empowered to act. It was not enough to recognize and say what we believe—we had to have a plan to act as well. By acting, we are supporting one another.

In keeping with the Mayo Clinic code of conduct and our pledge to always put the patient first and to uphold the Mayo Clinic values (respect, integrity, compassion, healing, teamwork, innovation, excellence, and stewardship), we committed as leaders to exhibit the following behaviors:

1. Show up as an aligned and coordinated leadership body with one voice.

2. Agree to respectfully give and receive authentic feedback.

3. Assume positive intent, approaching situations with curiosity.

4. Own and acknowledge when we do not hold to these commitments and address them in the venue where this occurred.

5. Foster a growth mindset by celebrating success and learning from failure.

6. Have one another's back and celebrate a circle of trust.

7. Validate others' feelings and perspectives with active listening.

8. Call out bystander behavior that is not actionable and not committed to change.

Good leaders intervene, correct, and respect their teams by giving them the gift of timely and specific behavioral feedback. Mastering the craft of giving feedback is the difficult part. Building an engaging vision and mission with team buy-in is a critical first step. Agreeing on the rules of play is a second. Amy Edmondson masterfully builds the case for this in her book *Extreme Teaming*, where she describes the elements essential to building a cohesive team, one that celebrates diversity of opinion, builds an engaging vision, cultivates psychological safety, and develops shared mental models.[1] These fundamentals help prevent burnout, isolation, harassment, frustration, inefficiency, and loss of focus. The same concepts that help our teams stay focused on the patient help to build a framework for success. I have lived both extremes, and trust me—much greater joy at work comes from mastering a shared mental model.

Staff must have a clear idea of expectations, as well as systems in place to help manage those expectations. A nurse anesthetist, for example, knows that she will administer anesthesia and other medications and that she will take care of people who receive or are recovering from anesthesia. She should not be expected to pass instruments or bring in equipment, nor should she be asked to. If someone encroaches on her territory or treats her with disdain, there should be a body that addresses that behavior respectfully and promptly. Individual responsibility is of vital importance, as are guardrails and duties. Equally important is having structures in place to protect people when others may overstep their boundaries.

But not all boundaries are created equal. When I came on staff at Mayo in 2014 I was given a lot of information about the institution. I read it all cover to cover—mostly. I have to admit to skimming some pages, such as those concerning the dress code. I was always professional in how I presented myself, so I wasn't really worried—until the day I was written up for toe cleavage, of all things. I knew about wearing pantyhose, about not coming to work in open-toed shoes or pants that exposed an ankle, but it never occurred to me to ensure that the split between my first and second toes wasn't visible when I wore my ballet flats, something that has been named "toe cleavage." Lesson learned.

As arbitrary as these rules seem (pantyhose is no longer mandatory, by the way), there is a very good reason for the dress code.

The Mayo brothers, William and Charles, wanted to create a very specific atmosphere for their patients. They worried that the standard white lab coat created distance between the physician and the patient, that it conveyed a sterile atmosphere that appeared to emphasize science over patient care. Most people have heard of the phenomenon called "white coat hypertension," a condition in which a patient's blood pressure rises simply from being at the doctor's office. We've tried to get around that by putting the patient first, and that includes considering the patient's feelings. Sure, everything we do at Mayo is powered by science, education, and research. That's a given. But nobody should feel like they're only a diagnosis or a list of symptoms. Putting the patient first is the cornerstone of support, something the Mayo brothers surely realized when they began practicing medicine at their father's clinic in the 1880s.

But as is often the case with protocols such as dress codes, they can hit one group disproportionately—in this case, women. Form-fitting dresses aren't allowed, for example, which is why I'll wear a blazer over any dress that might be deemed too snug. Leggings too, aren't permitted. I understand how they could be considered too casual, but I also think there should be some leeway, depending on individual circumstances. A colleague of mine recently had surgery and was wearing leggings because the compression helped ease her discomfort. Someone reported her for being in violation of dress and decorum, and she was written up and called in for counseling— even though she had a note from her own doctor recommending the leggings. (Even that, by the way, seemed infantilizing, as if this revered professional should have had to bring in a note from home.) The administrator and the doctor had an uncomfortable conversation and eventually the situation was resolved, but my colleague struggled over this for a long time. She lost confidence. Humiliated, she started to feel unable to be herself and worried about how people saw her. She felt uncomfortable in her own skin. Of Hispanic origin and a woman in medicine, she felt the target being drawn on her back. Why hadn't someone just mentioned the leggings to her directly, in a kind way? It would have saved so much time and energy. She never knew who reported her—*What was the psychology at work there?* she wondered—and she lost trust in her colleagues for a very long time. This kind of thing disproportionately happens to women physicians.

I'm proud to work at Mayo, but like so many institutions that have a long and storied legacy, it sometimes feels the burden of its history. These rules were likely published to create a professional atmosphere where everyone felt respected. We have patients from all over the world, some of whom might be offended by more relaxed Western attitudes toward what we consider to be appropriate attire. We've since done what we can to strike a happy medium on the dress code and behavior in general. I for one am happy that these old standards are no longer in place.

I'm a rule follower from way back, so while I respect and adhere to regulations, I also think it's important to reevaluate protocols from time to time. But it's not just the rules themselves, it's the way they are enforced. Rules should never take the place of respect, but, sad to say, sometimes that happens. It was my friend's experience that made me realize that we could do with more upstander training.

Mayo is very good at a great many levels of training—diversity, effective communication, and emotional intelligence. There's a mutual respect policy, an anti-retaliation policy, and a nondiscrimination policy. But like many hospitals, we're slow to understand what it means to be an upstander. Each part of the country has culturally different ways of working. The midwestern circuitous communication style can be difficult for both northerners and southerners to adapt to.

Ann Thompson is an upstander. A nurse practitioner who works in general internal medicine and has been around Mayo for a long time, she understands the patient population and how best to serve them. Ann goes above and beyond for her patients. She does what she can to make each one feel comfortable and to help them understand their treatment plan and follow-up care. When asked what she would like to be different about her job, she answered quickly: "More time with patients." But she understands the constraints we all work under, and does her best—always—to make sure that each patient feels respected and listened to. Still, things go wrong.

Over the past decade or so, Ann has noticed a difference in how people act and react when they're at the reception desk and sometimes even in the exam room. "There are more microaggressions coming from patients these days. They'll be disrespectful and oftentimes inappropriate. Not as much to providers, because there's a power differential there, but I've certainly seen people act out at receptionists and clerks when things don't go the way they expect.

"More than once I've had to step in and say, 'You know, gosh, I'm sorry that you had to wait, but your outburst is inappropriate, and we can't have you being disrespectful to our office staff.'"

Ann wasn't familiar with the term "upstander" until I brought it up to her. But she was the perfect example of one, someone who stands up for others. We need more of that.

There was a time in my career when I was given a new leadership opportunity and I felt tremendous responsibility. I wanted to make sure that I built my teams the way I had played things out in my head. I had gotten some negative feedback from a team member that I could be intimidating, and I wanted to work on that. I asked for a coach. Working with my coach, we went through the book *Crucial Conversations*.[2] That book taught me that it's not about winning an argument, getting your way, or even navigating politically difficult conversations; rather, it's about stepping into the shoes of another and understanding their perspective. When one person makes a comment in a meeting, everyone in the room has a different perspective and interpretation of how that comment lands. Some might be offended, while others are encouraged or even empowered. Sometimes the greatest lessons can be learned by having someone teach or show you another's perspective in a nonjudgmental way.

Feedback is a gift. The people who give feedback care. We are all imperfect humans. We could all use a little more forgiveness and a little less judgment. Being vulnerable and having a growth mindset with a willingness to learn can defuse many of the most volatile situations in life. Leaders must learn to advocate for and see the perspective of those who are without power and those who remain involuntarily vulnerable. They must spend time listening to the perspectives of the people they represent and discover how to ignite that fire in the belly that can drive a human to do amazing and visionary work. Great leaders know how to give feedback while at the same time making a person feel safe and inspired to do better.

Thirteen

The Myth of Work-Life Balance

Medical school is grueling. You go full tilt, in a routine that's all work and no play. The days are a haze of immunology, microbiology, physiology, pathology, and pharmacology. Apart from the -ologies, there are electives, clinical rotations, and, of course, residency. It's punishing and rewarding, a heady ride of highs and lows in which you push yourself to the extreme and are often physically and mentally exhausted. You long for time off, a simple dinner party or a night out with friends where you can engage with familiar faces and relax. But it's not as easy as you think. When you finally do go out, you feel like you're in a different world, looking at everything through a pane of glass. That's certainly how it was for me. I would show up for social events, but in reality, I was barely there—battling exhaustion as I tried to fit in with the rest of the crowd, a vague smile plastered on my face.

I remember one big occasion in 1994, when I was in the middle of medical school. I had just become engaged to my then boyfriend, Matt, now my husband of nearly thirty years, and his parents were throwing us an engagement party. I don't know if you've ever been to a party in Houston, but like everything else in Texas, the social events are oversized. This one at my future in-laws' home would be no exception.

I had a blast meeting more of Matt's family and friends—his aunts Becky and Bibi, who still lived in a small south Alabama town called Eufaula, and his uncle Herbert, a basketball coach whose claim to fame was recruiting Charles Barkley. I must have been told a hundred times by the Alabama crowd what a great basketball player Herbert had been back in the day. I remember bad boy Roy, Roy Dickson—the man whose face was bright red ten minutes into the party, not from drinking but from too much laughter. And I could never forget Roberta, who wore bright blue contacts and dramatic eyeliner. Back then, it was a look that was considered stunning, and she wore it well. Everyone seemed exaggerated and larger than life, a fun reminder that we weren't in Atlanta anymore. This was Texas.

I was having a wonderful time, but even though I tried to pace myself, as it got near my bedtime, which was typically 9:00 p.m., I started to droop. That's when I hit a wall of exhaustion. I was not just sleepy but the sort of bone-tired you get when staying upright is a challenge, when your body is sending you a message: *Bed. Now.* I held off for as long as I could, but by 10:00 p.m. I was sound asleep at the foot of the grand staircase, oblivious to the stares and whispers. One of the best survival tactics I learned in medical school and residency was "eat when you can, sleep when you can." I championed that and was well known for being able to sleep anywhere when I was tired enough. That day, I was tired enough . . . and then some.

"Matt, dear, is Shanda all right? Bless her heart . . ."

"Um, you do know that your fiancée is passed out, right?"

Matt took it all in stride. "This is the woman I'm marrying," he said. "She is definitely not intoxicated. This is who she is. She is either on or off. She works hard and gets exhausted. She goes to bed at nine and wakes at four a.m. almost every day. There's no middle ground. You'll get used to it."

A couple of times a year, I'm asked to give a talk on work-life balance. I always laugh when the topic comes up because, really, there is no such thing. I still give the talk, but I make it clear that this balance is as mythical as a unicorn, so don't bother trying to chase it. I like to put my own spin on the subject, speaking not about balance (the idea that you can reach an equilibrium between your personal and professional life) but about focus. Where and how you choose to spend your time, and specifically what you choose *not* to do, says a lot about how you balance yourself. Everyone's balance is different—there is no right or wrong.

I struggle to comprehend how hospitals and institutions provide adequate support for every person who works there when there is such disparity of effort and productivity. For example, a surgeon who does a small number of cases and rarely engages in research or other work activities might not need the same level of support as a practice partner who chooses to do a greater number of cases, more complex cases, and participate more heavily in research. In most institutions, though, they get the same level of support staff. This provides a disincentive for people to commit to extra work if it is not accompanied by additional support staff or protected time. The older and wiser me understands this more readily than my younger self did.

Our time here on earth is limited. As Oliver Burkman observed in his book *Four Thousand Weeks,* in which he lays out the ground rules for managing that time, "The average human lifespan is absurdly, insultingly brief. Assuming you live to be eighty, you have just over four thousand weeks."[1] Given this transience, focus seems to me to be an even more important attribute than balance, and a much better goal. Whereas balance encourages us to go after an evenness and constancy that seem always to be beyond our grasp, focus recognizes that we are not always going to have the same center of interest, that the object of our attention is going to change. What shouldn't change is our commitment to our profession and family. Life is too short to stay in a place that does not nurture us. That nurturing had better be constant, because without it we'll be lost.

Even throwing out that unattainable notion of elusive work-life balance, I often struggle with whether to encourage other women to enter the field. Thinking about some of the things I had to endure—not to mention the things my family has had to endure—I might not recommend it. It's hard to be a woman in a specialty dominated by men; that's why female-centric organizations like Women in Thoracic Surgery (WTS) are so meaningful. With a goal of sponsoring, mentoring, and supporting one another, the members hold each other up in a way that no one else can. We also complain together and commiserate. By feeling heard and understood, we give each other wise counsel and sponsorship. Being present in a place where you can be open and honest with others who think and feel the way you do holds tremendous value, no matter who you are. Minority groups find value in gathering with those who understand them and know them. This is basic. Just like esophageal cancer survivors find value in being among other survivors of the same illness, so do those with other struggles. It feels good to be understood.

When I first attended one of the WTS meetings, I found a group of around ten women surgeons having coffee in a small room lamenting the state of women in our specialty. It was an intimidating scene. They were giants in our specialty, and these women had accomplished so much already, including paving the way for women like me. In spite of that, I didn't realize how disappointed so many of them were. Specifically, they were complaining about how they got passed over for promotion, how their opportunities were limited, and how their experience was blunted by the fact that they were women. They told horror stories of how they had been treated and recounted comments by male surgeons, such as "You don't have to de-air the cannula if it is a woman" (meaning women are airheads, so trying to get the air out of the bypass pump is futile). Other comments included a man saying to one of my colleagues: "There are two kinds of women surgeons—those women who shouldn't be called surgeons and those women surgeons who shouldn't be called a woman."

That's changing now. With more and more women entering the field, we are rising through the ranks, effecting change, and getting more respect. That's much easier to do now that we have just as many women as men in residency and more than three hundred women are board-certified. The growth I have witnessed has led me to believe the existence of the WTS has brought meaning and value. It has to some degree sustained me when other groups did not.

As for that career path, no one can make that decision for another. We all take our own journeys, and no two are alike. That said, when a young woman asks me about entering the field, in addition to talking about the skills required and the long hours—and the incredible high you get when you help someone—I'll make sure to ask her what sort of support system she has in her life. Because life can be very difficult without an adequate one. I also tell her you don't go off-roading in rough terrain and expect a smooth ride. You have to be able to tolerate the bumps along your route.

Thank goodness I have a supportive husband to share my path. My husband has always taken my side, supported me, and stood by me. In the darkest of times, he has refused to leave me alone for fear of me falling off the cliff. He has molded his life to accommodate mine and my dreams—at the expense of his own.

Both Matt and I are children of divorce, so before we said "I do," we had some very long talks about what we wanted in our marriage and in our family. Scared of commitment, we both understood that to avoid the incredible losses associated with divorce—for ourselves and our kids—we would need to establish a means of speaking to each other and working through our marriage. For two years, Matt and I went for premarital counseling with our pastor, Dr. Jim Collins, of Peachtree Christian Church in Atlanta. (As the author of the book *Always a Wedding,* he seemed like a qualified candidate.)[2] The counseling was intense, but it was necessary to build a strong foundation and set ground rules.

Some of the rules were familiar: never letting the sun set on an argument, not fighting about things that happened in the past, and giving 100 percent each, instead of 50/50. Then there was the advice my stepfather, Tommy Bagwell, gave me: "To avoid a misunderstanding, you have to have an understanding." I believe this might be some of the best advice I have ever heard.

In sessions with our pastor, he encouraged us to focus on building trust, communication, and respect. He would repeat back to us what he heard, sometimes laughing at our comments, such as the time Matt and I asked him to review a marriage contract that we had drawn up. "Dr. Jim Collins, I would like to add a clause that says, 'Shanda will not involve my mom in any argument.' I don't want them ganging up on me for the rest of my life." (Kay did have a habit of taking my side.)

I'm not sure Matt knew what he was getting into when he married me. I certainly didn't have any idea of the realities of balancing marriage, motherhood, and surgery. Sometimes it feels like the most natural thing in the world. After several hours in surgery, I'll come home to my family and we'll share stories about the day, maybe build a fire in the fireplace, and settle under a cozy blanket with a movie and some popcorn. I'll feel grateful beyond measure and fulfilled. Then there are the times when it feels as if I'm juggling chainsaws. Some nights I feel like the hospital ate me for dinner and I am bringing the table scraps of myself home to my family. I strive to be a dedicated parent, just as I strive to be a dedicated surgeon. But oftentimes there's a clash.

The raw truth is that I often have to prioritize my patients and specialty above my family and children. When I missed my son Jake's music recital because I had to remove a cancer, that was justified. There was never any question of what I had to do, but I regret missing the big event. When I asked how I could make it up to him, he suggested we have our own concert. I came home and walked into the basement to find him ready to play his viola. This precious child of mine had been practicing at school all of this time—away from my view—and proceeded to blow me away with one of my favorite songs, "Hallelujah" by Leonard Cohen. It was beautiful, so haunting and full of love. I was still sad at not having been in the school auditorium, at not having been able to sit in the audience and beam along with the other proud parents, but I felt something else, a sense of pride at the young man I was raising—talented, yes, and also compassionate. It wasn't the same as being there for him, but I take comfort that he knew how much I cared. We found a lot of compromises and unique ways to show our love while I was deeply engaged in this all-consuming career.

Life is full of difficult decisions, and when we care for one another we are able to find a place to meet in the middle that may even be better than what we imagined. My not being there for my son was tough, but I took the opportunity to explain why I was absent and how fortunate I was to be able to make a difference in someone else's life. I did my best to help him navigate his disappointment (and mine), and maybe teach him something in the process. Having Jake understand the world as a complex place (and learn that he's not always at the epicenter) was a valuable lesson. That doesn't mean I don't have moments of weakness when I want to give up everything and focus on my family. There are days when I straddle my feelings of wanting to be a good mother and wanting to be a good surgeon, days when I know I can't be both. Sometimes I feel like this is something I'm doing for myself and I feel selfish, like the two things I want to do in this world couldn't be further away from each other. But other times I realize how many people I'm helping (more than 7,000 patients so far) and that my presence in the OR really does make a difference.

∿

When you don't have your squad lined up, when you don't have a strong home base, everything is more difficult. My marriage isn't perfect. My husband and I have our ups and downs like everybody else, but having a shared understanding and a mutual respect goes a long way. As does having shared goals and, frankly, a tacit agreement to support each other, no matter what. It's not easy being a doctor's spouse. It never has been.

Way back in 1979, the *New York Times* published an article entitled "Doctors' Wives: Many Report Marriage Is a Disappointment."[3] "The time and energy demands of the medical profession were seen as taking a terrible toll on a doctor's family," the article states. One woman, who was married to a doctor for a great many years, commented, "My husband's patients always came first and still do!" The article cited resentment, a failure to compromise, and the need to be a supportive spouse "without much emotional support or positive feedback" as the drawbacks of being married to someone within the medical profession. They are always late for dinner, their pagers go off during movies, they fall asleep in the middle of conversations, they don't shut off when they get home.

That the spouses interviewed by the *Times* were all women is a reflection of the piece being written more than forty years ago. The demographic makeup has changed substantially since then. In 1980, women made up less than 10 percent of physicians.[4] In 2019 that figure was 36 percent.[5] While we are only 6 percent of my specialty, what hasn't changed are the demands of the medical profession. They certainly haven't subsided. Some may argue that they have even increased, as many doctors feel they are being pressured to be part of a healthcare machine, rather than a healthcare team. Burdened with administrative details, they are driven further away from their families, as they now stay late after work getting all of the electronic health records work done, held hostage to online ratings by patients and Press Ganey survey scores with little forgiveness for being human.

As a medical professional, you are committed to science and humanity. You are dedicated to giving your patients and their families the best care you can. But sometimes that dedication takes its toll, and you are the one who needs help. Sometimes you need to look for higher ground, a place where you can disconnect from your responsibilities, recharge, and be with the ones you love. A place where you can truly be understood. Because without it, and without people who will support you unconditionally, you may be lost.

That's what happened to one of my best friends. She tried to do it all without any help from her husband. She worked as a surgeon, but also took care of the kids and managed all of the finances. He drank too much and simply went to work and came home, where he did nothing. Her life was as miserable as her husband was. We would talk on the phone and discuss options. Her job suffered, as she barely had the energy to drive to work. When one of her workplace colleagues began to bully her, it tipped her over the edge. Her leader took the side of the bully because they'd been partners and friends in a lab prior to the current job. Alas, this is far too common. Finally she gathered the strength to separate from and later divorce both her workplace and her husband. But that led to losing custody of her children. It almost destroyed her.

Far too often we are held together by a thin thread; it doesn't take very much to unravel the entire thing. She had no support other than a few friends and her parents. I worried she might take her life. I fretted that she would find it impossible to manage life changes. Slowly, though, she began to rebuild her life piece by piece. Much of her recovery can be attributed to joining a physician support group led by the legendary Dr. Mike Maddaus, a physician life coach, and to connecting with friends in a meaningful way. We held her up and supported her. We helped her see her worth, understand her path, and move toward something bigger and better. It turns out that we can be rescued, but it takes a very strong support network, routine connection, sometimes psychiatric care, sometimes prayer, sometimes periods of time away from work, and always a lot of active listening.

We all take turns. An almost equal number of times, my friend has supported me. We call each other early in the morning before we leave for work and solve problems together on the phone, navigating and listening to one another. We are our own support for one another. She has helped me weather more than just one storm.

Fourteen

Complications

I will never forget my first patients, nor will I forget the doctors and staff I have worked with over the years. As I was finishing up my time in Houston, I noticed one of my partners attempting more advanced and complicated surgeries. Specifically, Tom was trying to remove the pancreas laparoscopically through small incisions, guided by a camera inside the body. This is called a laparoscopic Whipple (pancreatectomy). This is minimally invasive surgery—tiny ports are placed into the abdomen, carbon dioxide is used to inflate the abdomen like a dome, and then small stick-shaped instruments are used to perform the surgery)—and it's one of the most difficult surgeries in the world to perform well. Working around critically large vessels, moving bowels, and navigating the biliary tree are difficult under any circumstances, and the vast amount of "cutting and pasting" needed to remove a pancreas can be overwhelming, even when the patient's abdomen is open in front of the surgeon. But performing a laparoscopic Whipple is like eating rice with chopsticks underwater with a shark swimming around.

Not many people were doing minimally invasive pancreatectomies in 2013. Many of us wanted to learn difficult maneuvers and push the envelope with minimally invasive surgery, but we also wanted to put our patients first, doing it slowly with careful observation and mentorship, making sure we had excellent outcomes. This is one of the paradoxes in modern surgery. We want to adopt new procedures to help our patients, but there's always a learning curve, and we worry that patients on the early part of that curve may pay the price. This is exactly why patients are taught to ask surgeons how many times they have performed a particular procedure, to try and eliminate the probability of being on the early part of that learning curve.

Because it's important to reduce bad outcomes, hospitals perform analyses and conduct events like the morbidity and mortality conference. The M&M conference is an in-house forum where complications are presented and decisions, actions, and responses are discussed. It's an opportunity to evaluate procedures and the surgeons who perform them. These conversations are meant for learning, introspection, and self-improvement, which is why residents also attend. Today, we record all cases, and when something goes wrong we play back the video so that we can learn from our mistakes. Often when I give a lecture I will include a video of my missteps, describing my error and how I fixed the problem. This sort of transparency and open learning is vital to a growth mindset, which is the belief that a person's capacities and talents can improve over time.

That's not the only means of dealing with residents or surgeons who have made questionable decisions or have had bad outcomes. There's also a quality committee that monitors surgeons who are at risk of going astray, watching their progress and patient interactions. This committee can also be linked to risk management when legal issues come up, thereby raising the stakes for the doctor and hospital alike. Then there is each state's board of medical examiners, to which practitioners are reported when things get out of hand or hospitals do a poor job of helping their doctors stay safe.

The morbidity and mortality conference and the quality committee are vital in ensuring patient safety. They hold physicians and surgeons accountable for their actions and identify adverse outcomes associated with medical error. These conferences and committees seek to modify behavior and fine-tune judgment based on experience, in order to prevent future errors and the complications that arise from them. Yet as necessary as these conferences and committees are, they are also incredibly intimidating. Gathering surgical staff inside a conference room to highlight cases, discuss mistakes, and focus on areas of potential improvement in the way patients receive care can be nerve-racking. Patient events are a serious matter and should be discussed in an open forum. However, the trauma that often ensues after a surgeon makes a mistake frequently never gets dealt with, and that's a problem.

A well-run M&M conference isn't judgmental. It doesn't seek to ostracize or shame surgeons. But it doesn't aim to support them either. That's a problem. I have never felt personally judged at an

M&M conference, but I have spoken to colleagues who have felt the stress of presenting a difficult case only to feel that the people gathered in the room weren't on their side. That instead of looking for ways to improve the situation, they were looking for ways to build a case against them. Although anything discussed at an M&M conference is considered privileged and confidential, much of the information nevertheless ends up being discussed in the hallways and locker room after the meeting. That can put the surgeon in a compromising and vulnerable position.

Surely there's a better way to support each other, to find out why things take a wrong turn and what we can do to avoid similar outcomes in the future. Since teamwork and professionalism are something we all aspire to, I like to ask for input from team members at the end of surgery, and borrow the debriefing process from the Blue Angels model, a concept introduced by a colleague of mine whom I respect and admire, Dr. Joe Dearani. The US Navy's Blue Angels, a flight demonstration squadron formed just after World War II, whose mission is to showcase the teamwork and profes- sionalism of the Navy and Marine Corps, have a systematic format they go through after every mission, in which the team regroups to candidly discuss the details of what happened, what worked well, and what could be done better. What's more, they always end with a humble "glad to be here" expression of gratitude.

I sometimes think that we in the medical profession don't stop long enough to really look at our errors and to consider the potential improvements we might make. We might be running between two operating rooms, doing rounds, answering emails, doing research, and working on too many other things. Anyone can find you anywhere now; you cannot even go to the bathroom without your pager going off. Your day is consumed by all the people who need you, people who are unaware of the competitors for your attention. Because we are pulled in so many directions, we become defensive and we begin to lose sight of the gift of a simple task or a simple moment. So having the type of structured conversations that occur in an M&M conference or a quality committee meeting allows us the opportunity to pause and reflect, to open ourselves to comment. Because we are inviting the feedback, we are less defensive. It forces us to take an essential break for the more important things.

Much has been written about "the surgeon's personality." Among the traits associated with this profession are high levels of determination, focus, and conscientiousness. A study published in *The Surgeon: Journal of the Royal Colleges of Surgeons of Edinburgh and Ireland*[1] found that, in general, surgeons and surgical residents scored lower on neuroticism and higher on conscientiousness and extroversion than those in the general population. But neuroticism—which typically means that a person is more likely than average to experience anxiety, worry, fear, anger, guilt, depressed mood, and loneliness—increases as surgeons get older. Not just that, but the study cited "the high workload and relatively higher and prolonged exposure to morbidity and mortality in patients, and emotional situations" as among the reasons for that increase in neuroticism. Substance abuse, instability at home, and relationship problems only compound these issues.

Having a supportive team, strong mentors, and understanding leadership, not to mention friends, can help soften the blows and prevent someone from succumbing to the dark side. Unfortunately, at a time when my Houston partner Tom's work was challenging, his personal life was also becoming more complicated. Often these things are related. Tom was pushing the boundaries of medicine and surgery at the same time he was falling in love. It was a head-over-heels type of relationship that seemed to eclipse everything. With this heady combination of new love and new work, the world was his oyster. Until it wasn't. It all came to an end when my partner had a very public breakup with his fiancée, and that damaged his reputation.

Having one of the brightest minds I have ever encountered, and being equipped with what most would call a photographic memory, Tom could have been anything. But a brilliant mind alone is not a predictor of success, especially when it comes to surgery. One spiral led to another, and fast. When you don't feel good at home, your work can suffer. And not feeling good at work can affect your home life. My spouse, Matt, can attest to that. Whenever I have a difficult time at the clinic, he says that the family feels it too. He also notes that on operating days, which are often some of my best days, everyone at home says they can tell I was operating that day because of the good mood it puts me in and the smile on my face when I walk in the door.

Unfortunately for Tom, the notoriety that resulted from the quarrel with his fiancée cost him patients, time, and money, not to mention his pride. I could see the toll this was taking on him. Tom started to show signs of depression. He began coming into work late, missing clinics, not showing up for scheduled surgeries, and isolating himself from his colleagues. What's more, complications during his surgeries, previously rare for this surgeon, were happening more and more often. His favorite nurse left his practice. His fiancée was gone and suing him for defamation. His world seemed to be crumbling around him.

I had seen it before. The pattern was clear. Lost dream, lost trust, lost support. So much loss.

When I had been in general surgery residency in Atlanta, one of my friends suffered a head injury, the result of a car accident sustained while driving home one night after a long shift at the hospital. Many people have stories of driving drowsy, most of them being near misses. But this accident was devastating. Peter was in med school in Augusta but was doing some of his clinical rotations with us in Atlanta. This meant a lot of road travel.

Sleep deprivation is real among physicians, an all-too-common experience with sometimes tragic results. Peter fell asleep and his car collided with a bridge column; the impact caused bleeding into my friend's brain, leaving him with a movement disorder and cutting short his career as a surgeon, which requires absolutely steady hands. Yet, somehow, the accident didn't affect his intellect. None of us ever doubted that he was smart enough to take care of very sick patients. He could even place lines and catheters in spite of his movement disorder, a result of damage to the basal ganglia. But surgery was out.

Devastated at losing the professional future he had long worked toward, Peter turned to critical care to find a fulfilling career path. But the long nights involved in that specialty took a toll. Plus everything changed for him as a result of his movement disorder, awkward way of walking, and exaggerated facial expressions, which all stemmed from the injuries he had incurred—and that's to say nothing of the pain, which pushed Peter to opioid use.

Unfortunately, substance abuse in the healthcare profession is a growing problem. "Physicians are invested with awesome responsibility and trust. We are thought of as invulnerable, as miracle workers, and we're told, 'Heal thyself.' We're no better at that than the rest of you and in some ways, we're far worse," says Peter Grinspoon, a primary care physician in Boston and an instructor at Harvard Medical School.[2] Physicians who struggle often don't seek help, as doing so may affect their medical reputation and ability to obtain a medical license. Professional counseling means mandated reporting on most medical license applications and renewals, which means that any effort you make to formally heal yourself might lead to your losing your ability to practice medicine. Because of this, physicians often try to hide it all and treat or heal themselves.

I worried about my friend. I didn't know at the time that he had a substance abuse issue, but based on his absences from work and his increasingly negative attitude, I was worried something was up. As the days went on, he showed up for work later and later. It seemed possible that whatever he was doing at night was spilling into the day. But because he had a movement disorder, it was impossible to tell if he was intoxicated. No one smelled alcohol on his breath, nor did we see him consuming drugs or alcohol. Nevertheless, it was clear he was struggling.

I did my best to stay close to Peter. He assured me that everything was fine. The only thing he mentioned was that he was having trouble making it to the doctor for follow-up for his brain injury. He asked me if I would renew his prescription for Coumadin, a blood thinner used to prevent blood clots. Peter showed me the old script and told me that he had to stay on it because of "cavernous sinus thrombosis." A blood clot inside your brain is a serious problem, and I didn't want him to die because he'd missed his doctor's appointment, so I agreed. I wish I could have done more than just call the pharmacy on his behalf.

When Peter's depression worsened, when his mood became darker, I reached out to his family. I told them that he was markedly depressed and might be in trouble, that he might harm himself. I had hoped for compassion and concern but was met with denial and exasperated silence, then defensive accusations. I didn't know what I was talking about, they told me. Shouldn't I mind my own business rather than sticking my nose in where it didn't belong?

I was at a loss as to what to do. Had I made things worse? Would my interference push my friend even further down into the pit of depression?

My worst fears were realized when one day Peter didn't show up for work. Again I called to check on him. I left messages. I called over and over before I eventually went to my chiefs and asked them to go to his apartment. They heard no answer when they knocked, but there was a shuffling and scraping sound that alarmed them. It turned out he had barricaded himself in the apartment. They unsuccessfully tried to force the door open, unsuccessfully tried to get a key, and finally called the fire department to break the door in. As the door opened, Peter shot himself in the head with a handgun. Unlike the many patients we cared for who attempted suicide that way but missed and instead were wounded, my friend's aim was clear and accurate. He died in front of our chiefs.

It was this image that coursed through me years later as everything was playing out with my partner Tom. I told myself I would not let this happen again. This time, I knew the signs. This time, I was going to do better.

I called Tom. I called and called. No answer. I went to his home, where I found his dogs tied outside the door. They looked like they'd been there for a while. Had they been fed? Did they have enough water? There was dog poop everywhere and the porch was filthy. Tom loved his dogs, and he was also obsessively neat. This made me worry. Distraught, I banged on the door. No one came.

I was aware of what could happen, but because I had suspected he might be in trouble and read about ways to intervene, because I reached out, I thought I could make a difference. I wasn't the only one. He had other friends who were there for him, who tried to throw him a lifeline. We all tried to help. We all thought that by talking to Tom—and listening—he might find a way out of the darkness.

Thankfully, he realized the dire position he was in and, admitting that he needed help, got himself to rehab. After intensive treatment, he thought he could return to his job. He tried to come back but was fired. The unforgiving nature of the medical profession made it almost impossible for him to continue to practice medicine.

Having practiced as a brilliant surgeon, trained residents, and held offices in national leadership organizations, Tom couldn't cope with the world he found himself in. No support group existed. Who do you turn to when your brilliant future is cut short? How do you go on? Tom needed to work. Not just for the money, but for the sense of self-respect. He was a smart man, dedicated to medicine and to his patients. One wrong move led to another, and soon it seemed that nobody would help him.

Tom and I kept in touch, texting and talking on the phone. I was feeling better about his prospects once he had gone through rehab. He wasn't quite the old Tom I knew—and that might not have been a bad thing—but he seemed on the way to something better. Our conversations seemed to give him hope, and I naively thought I was helping him by giving him a way to vent and heal.

When he told me that he had become engaged to his girlfriend and they were expecting a child, I heard a lightness in his voice. I still remember walking with my son to baseball practice and talking on the phone with Tom as I dragged the Radio Flyer wagon full of baseball equipment and snacks to the nearby baseball field. Tom and I were trying to find a night to have dinner together and arguing good-naturedly about where we would go. He wanted me to meet his fiancée, and he said he would bring her over to the house for dinner. He texted me a photograph of them in Mexico together—their faces were so beautiful and relaxed. Healing seemed to be taking place in spite of the deep scars.

But he spoke about having to work taking histories and doing physical exams at an urgent care center. It was mundane work, and it did nothing to gratify him. He expressed anger over being fired from his job. He felt abandoned. He wanted to be back working at the hospital with us. He wanted to be financially stable, to have his patients back, and to have the internet stories about him erased.

I mistakenly detected healing and hope in Tom's voice, perhaps because I wanted it to be there. The memory of Peter still haunted me, and his ghost continued to hover whenever I spoke to Tom. Our talk ended as I arrived at the ballfield and my son began demanding money for a snow cone. Just before hanging up, I broke my big news: I had accepted a position at Mayo Clinic. Tom muttered something about me being "the last rat to jump ship." He laughed a little, maybe picturing that original group of bright and energetic surgeons who thought they were going to change the world from the 16th floor of the Smith building.

We promised to speak again soon, but I felt awkward as we ended our call. I could imagine how he must have felt, working so hard yet still facing so many hurdles. I felt for him, but there was no denying that I was excited to work for an institution with the motto "The patient always comes first." I was so thrilled to join an organization that was run by physicians, rather than administrators who had never held the life of a human being in their hands, that I gave up my post as chief of my division and actually took a pay cut. I wanted the opportunity to expand my research with resources that were limitless and work with colleagues who would teach me. In many ways it felt like a dream come true. And yet I couldn't help but feel uncomfortable knowing that I was on a good pathway and my friend was not.

Tom and I texted back and forth after that. Then, on the night before we moved to Rochester, when I was in a random hotel room in Denver because of a canceled United Airlines flight, my daughter asleep in my lap, a friend called to tell me of his death. The same path, the same spiral. The same devastation and loss. Again.

Fifteen

Provider Support

My first days at Mayo were filled with silent tears. Apart from the ladies' room, there was no private place to cry. I signed myself up for counseling to try to find a way to deal with the grief and guilt I felt at my friend's death. I tried to understand what happened, how loss of hope had led to despair and how that, in turn, had led to substance abuse. From there it was a dramatic pull, a spiral that led to more loss of hope, disconnection from support, and finally death.

Watching someone go from being on top of the world as a great teacher and surgeon, financially stable, and with a great reputation to being dismissed by his profession, shunned by his community, and ultimately bankrupt—that was one of the worst spirals I have ever witnessed. It made me realize that, as I said earlier, far too often we are held together only by a thin thread. Our lives may feel solid, but they are fragile and can easily unwind. Without tremendous support from our community, that unraveling can deliver even the strongest of us to the grave.

My arrival at Mayo Clinic should have been a happy time for me and my family. We were all starting a new life, embarking on a new adventure. However, after learning of my friend's death, leaving all of my patients behind in Houston, and saying goodbye to my in-laws, who lived down the street and helped us daily, we arrived in a completely different climate. Aside from some vague familiarity with my new partners, we knew no one. We learned how isolating it can be to live among reserved midwesterners, whose demeanor can often be cool, much like the climate they live in—and very unlike the South. I love Minnesota and have so many friends here now, but it wasn't so easy in the beginning. It was a whole different way of life for all of us. It wasn't just learning to say "pop" instead of "soda," or getting used to the expression "you betcha." Unlike our neighborhood in Houston, where we had forty-five children on the block, all playing inside and outside our homes and running between houses, the people in our new neighborhood were more mature. Most of the children had graduated from college, and their parents were in a different phase of life. We had to slowly learn to rebuild the community of friends we needed to survive.

While we settled in, I found myself incredibly sad about the loss of my friend. Perhaps I was too sad, as I seemed to focus on it several times each day. I traveled to his home and met with his sister and mother, giving them photographs that I had from our social gatherings. I stayed in touch with his fiancée, as she was expecting their child. The sadness was overwhelming, and my mixed emotions about this new place where I had brought my family began to evolve into doubt.

Had I made a mistake? Had I ruined the lives of my children by transplanting them here to the frozen tundra, leaving all of their friends behind? Before I accepted the job we'd made lists of pros and cons as a family, and we'd made the move only after we all agreed, after it became clear that I'd be able to regularly make it home at night to see the family—unlike in Houston, where I might go days without seeing the kids. I knew my time would be managed better at Mayo. I calculated that I could do twice as many cases as at my old hospital in half the time. Instead of every other night on call, I would instead take hospital calls one night out of six. My partners all said they were routinely home for dinner because of the efficiency. Living in Rochester, which despite a population of 120,000 felt like a small town, might make life simpler for my family. I thought my career would be better as well.

But had I really thought things through completely?

Ironically, one of the biggest losses I felt when I left Houston was the loss of my amazing secretary. Elaine had made all of my medical and personal appointments. She kept my life on track and made me look good. She made sure I got out of work to make it to the kids' school events. She noticed when my gray roots started showing and would make an appointment for a touch-up. She organized my minimally invasive surgery courses and knew every patient by first and last name. More importantly, she knew their stories. She was one of the most incredible partners in life I had ever had, and I'd forgotten to put her name on the list of pros and cons. I had underestimated the light she brought to my life every day. These micro-illuminations contributed more to my happiness than I realized. The personal relationships and support my local team from Houston had given me were overwhelmingly good. I had to try to find a way to build the same thing here in Rochester.

I went into the restroom to cry almost every day. I cried some days for the loss of my friend Tom. Some days I cried for the sadness of my children adjusting to our new life; I envisioned them coming off the school bus with tears running down their faces. Other days, I cried from the worry about whether I had done the right thing. Never did I question my ability to perform surgery or make decisions about patients. The things that brought me sadness and created worry were those more personal issues that affect us daily.

I often tell people that when bad things happen there's always some good that will come out of it. But I saw no good in this and had no way to process it. Here I was in a new job and a new city, without my support structure. The irony was that the patient support group in Houston had gotten me through hell, helping me hang on when I might have succumbed like the others. It reminded me of why I'd gone into my field, the impact I might have, and the true foundations of healthcare. The support group had given me so much. It was my compass and I felt lost without it. I had thought I was there to support them, but really they'd been supporting me. And now I was on my own.

Thinking of my colleagues who had died—and realizing that everyone there had a colleague who had died—I came to the conclusion that we had to do something. We had to stand up for one another. We had to get busy correcting the system to make it safer for us all, not just the patients. Held up by my team, my family, and the people I loved, I could endure. Take those away and I become vulnerable.

I was once again feeling as if I was to blame. But then I realized that there is a system that has driven so many bright, thoughtful, talented people to the grave, and there was a common theme. We have disconnected from one another, and we are left on our own at sea, with nothing to keep us afloat. Watching people drown one after the other made me think we were all going down, like we were sinking on the *Titanic*. We had to do something.

It was because of this that I submitted a proposal to Women in Thoracic Surgery to create a support group for women surgeons and initiated a wellness task force for the Society of Thoracic Surgeons. I was chair of the society's Council for Clinical Practice and Member Engagement, and we recruited members to run that task force, which evolved into a variety of initiatives to improve the lives of our surgeon colleagues. These teams have started meeting either officially or unofficially—whatever best suits their aims and schedules. I also helped to organize a physician engagement group here at Mayo Clinic. The Physician Engagement Group (PEG) is a group of female surgeons who lean on one another for support. I trust these women with my life. They have seen me through some very difficult times. We get together in a restaurant or in someone's home and talk about difficult cases and situations. There are rules, of course, the most important being that if you are discussing a patient who had a terrible outcome, it has to be *your* outcome. We don't confer about someone who's absent from the meeting, nor do we engage in rumors and gossip. Rules and guardrails are as important as a compass. You don't support one person by knocking down another.

I have had the privilege of being a member and sometimes leader of many organizations, such as Women in Thoracic Surgery, American Association for Thoracic Surgeons, Society of Thoracic Surgeons, American College of Surgeons, and Southern Thoracic Surgical Society. Each of these organizations has provided to some degree a resource, guidance, friendship, and comradery. Groups like these can sustain us and bring us joy. Most of the time, I feel that they're like a family by choice—strong but imperfect. We follow each other's careers and lives along the way from training to death. But cardiothoracic surgeons are competitive creatures, and sometimes these organizations can also serve to feed ugly parts of ourselves, like pride, ego, and greed. I've seen it all.

And then there is Mike Maddaus's book club, which has been a lifeline. I first heard of Mike when he was in Minneapolis working as a renowned thoracic surgery educator, funded researcher, and clinician—someone we called a "triple threat." At the University of Minnesota, he was responsible for training some of the brightest young minds in our field. By all accounts he was a wonderful leader. I learned of Mike because we were eager to recruit one of his young residents to our program when I was teaching for MD Anderson Cancer Center. From her, I heard about how he had cultivated her career and how he had inspired her to go into the field. I listened as she told me stories about what a positive influence he had been in her life. I felt good that she had such a strong and capable supporter. I may even have felt a little envious that I hadn't had someone like that when I was in the early stages of my career. This young woman was at the top of our rank list that year, so I couldn't blame her when she decided to stay in Minneapolis so that she could continue her work with him.

Unfortunately—tragically—several months after she matched in the program to train for thoracic surgery, Mike became addicted to prescription narcotics while recovering from a lumbar fusion and hip replacement. It was a very dark period for him, and today he talks openly about his struggles and how they led to the end of his surgical career. He speaks about how no one was allowed to contact him or reach out for three months while he was in treatment. He speaks about the isolation that comes from so rapidly falling from the top of the world into the pit of despair. But at the time, the rumor mill being what it is, I heard about his struggles, not from him but from a great many of my colleagues. And then I heard about the end of his career, and the usual swirl of gossip when one of us falls from grace.

Eventually the talk slowed down, and Mike went through rehabilitation and came out on the other side. He spent time as a stay-at-home father and husband caring for his family while his wife continued to work as a high-risk obstetrician. Once his children were grown, he reengaged in our specialty. Not as a surgeon this time, but as a coach full of life experience, insight, and raw honesty. He found strength in his vulnerability. This was something we had never seen in a cardiothoracic surgeon—humbleness, vulnerability, humanity. But it was a long road.

As Mike himself tells it, a devastating personal fall became a second chance. "We come into our medical world with the American culture kind of beaten into us. It's fortified and strengthened over the course of training and then our career. That idea of self-sufficiency is so deeply bred into us that asking for help feels like a weakness."

I listened intently as he told me this, because I knew all too well the pressures of perfection, the feeling that you always need to be strong, that you can't show any sort of vulnerability. The isolation born of this false narrative came roaring into my life with the onset of menopause, which for me was an excruciating experience. My body was changing. I felt extremes of temperatures—one minute the room was freezing and the next like an oven—causing me to sweat profusely in my operating gown during surgery. I also felt at times as if I was losing my mind. I became forgetful of things in a way I never was before, my sleep was disrupted, and I slept even less, if that was possible. These challenges leaked out to my colleagues, causing them to think I wasn't pulling my weight or keeping track of patients like I should. They complained that I needed too many reminders to check in on tests and follow up on routine matters.

Instead of compassion and understanding—instead of help—I got added pressure from my leadership. No one stopped for a split second to ask me how I was doing, what I was thinking, or what was going on.

I reached out for help to better understand what I was going through. I longed for guidance, for some way to self-correct. I used every resource available to me. But I continued to struggle with certain teams. It was a stressful time and I had to rescue myself. I went to the Women's Health Program at Mayo Clinic and started estrogen therapy. That helped greatly with my physical symptoms. Still, I felt separated from the pack. My colleagues and leaders were used to thinking of me as someone who had never taken a sick day, as someone who previously ran marathons and had boundless energy. They didn't know what to do when I appeared vulnerable. Menopause was debilitating. But the lack of awareness and compassion by my colleagues and leaders brought me to my knees.

Why did no one say how terrible this would be? Was it just me? Were other women surgeons struggling with this?

I leaned heavily on those who supported me. I cannot imagine how other female surgeons without such support deal with the emotional and physical turmoil. It made pregnancy with twins seem easy. I'm glad to be on the other side of this; however, so many of my friends are still in the mire.

I have since learned that our former CEO at Mayo, Dr. John Noseworthy, has taken on the health psycho-social challenges of women in menopause as a new career focus. I was so grateful to see such a strong and good leader attending to such a big problem. He has partnered with Upliv Health to build a new patient-centered model for providing menopause care in partnership with Northwell. Research shows ignoring menopause in the workplace widens the equity gap. Women in their forties and fifties are some of the most experienced managers, and overlooking their needs may come at a significant cost to everyone. With the aging US workforce, menopause is estimated to cost American women an estimated $1.8 billion in lost working time per year. Thank goodness someone is taking the initiative to address this.

Mike Maddaus would agree: "We need support, we need to talk to people, but when we keep denying the pain—maybe because we don't recognize what's going on . . . maybe because we're too damn busy to actually check in with ourselves—well, it's not a good situation." He talked to me further about his own experience, about how he never really reached out for support for any of his struggles and how a big part of that was the alchemy of being male as well as the inculcation of surgical culture. He concluded, "These habits of surgeons, like pretending you're okay when you're not, and self-sufficiency, you know . . . these are really valuable habits to have as a surgeon, when needed. But like everything, they are good until they aren't. Surgeons, and all humans really, make the mistake of thinking that because something brings success in one arena, that it applies to all walks of life. Not true."

Mike has come through the other side with profound insights on vulnerability and support. He has found peace with his struggles and is now using his own hard-earned lessons to support others. I admire that. I admire him, of course. So much so that I named him chief of the Society of Thoracic Surgeons Task Force on Wellness. STS represents approximately seven thousand cardiothoracic surgeons and is one of the biggest organizations to advocate for us as a whole. Since then, he has taken on this issue for our members with his usual intensity. A champion for wellness, he talks about the psychological consequences on the surgeon of making a serious medical or technical error, including the death of a patient.

He has written several powerful articles, two of which are "The Resiliency Bank Account" and "The Second Victim," which talks about what happens to a surgeon who loses a patient. He has a podcast called *The Resilient Surgeon* in addition to a support-group-style book club. He speaks at our annual meetings and works as a coach as well.

A friend of mine lost his wife a few years ago. As a leader in thoracic surgery, he had the world in front of him. Sadly, the grief he experienced sent him into a tailspin, landing him in a deep depression. Attempts at self-rescue failed. When he went to his leaders asking for assistance, he was told not to seek inpatient psychiatric counseling or any formal care because that requires mandatory disclosure and would go onto his record. The state medical board keeps track of physicians' mental health issues in such great detail that it can impair their ability to gain future employment. There is no privacy.

Mike Maddaus and I firmly believe this policy should be changed because of the effect it has on physicians who need to seek help. Instead of getting help, they avoid it to preserve their careers. Ironically, it does the exact opposite.

Fortunately, my friend who needed help had the wherewithal to leave the country and seek that help off the record. When he became strong enough to return to the United States, he still didn't deem himself fit enough to practice medicine again. Not yet, anyway. So, like Mike Maddaus, he sought refuge in family, retreating to a safe place by moving in with his kids and taking care of his grandchildren. My friend flourished in this environment. What an unexpected gift to be so close to those he loved. He enjoyed this precious time so much that he even made me think about doing the same, taking a year off and just being a stay-at-home parent. So many surgeons—male and female alike—have had the fantasy. His situation provided a unique opportunity to do something we all at one point in time had dreamed of. He's back at work now. I think that, as he slowly assimilates back into our world, he no doubt has a new and unique perspective.

I continue to work with STS to advocate for our members—and this includes attending the legislative advocacy workshop and lobbying Congress on behalf of our patients and our workforce on issues such as this. We have to find a better pathway to health. Telling surgeons that they can't seek mental health help is not the right answer. Through the wellness workforce, Mike and I will work to make sure the rest of the world knows that. I will continue to try to make things right and tell the stories of our colleagues and patients to anyone who will listen to our unique perspective.

The physician wellness program at Mayo Clinic has done incredible work to define the prevalence, causes, and consequences of physician burnout across the career span, developing evidence-based interventions that improve the work and lives of physicians as well as the care they provide patients. It evaluates the entire spectrum of personal, professional, and organizational factors that influence physician well-being, satisfaction, and productivity, researching optimal organizational approaches to prevent physician stress and working to create a positive energy workplace. We also have other, more creative programs, like the HELP Program, which is a peer support program for colleagues who've experienced stressful or traumatic work-related events. Mentorship programs, formal or informal, are available to help guide physicians over the course of their careers as well. Coaches are essential in helping physicians optimize their performance and define what brings them the most joy in their careers.

If there's one good thing that came out of the COVID-19 pandemic—as I said, I really do believe that when bad things happen some good will come out of it—it has been a focus on the importance of mental health. More people are willing to talk about anxiety and depression now. It's not the taboo it once was. And where there is dialogue, there can be hope. When we connect, we can pull each other through tough times and help prevent burnout and the depression that can come with it.

Sixteen

Managing Survivorship

Unlike at Houston Methodist, most of the patients at Mayo aren't local, which made an in-person support group impossible. I struggled to set up an environment similar to the one we had in Houston—an environment that would let me provide the best care for my patients and allow me to continue that care after they had been discharged from the hospital. But it wasn't easy.

Typically, patients who come into the clinic have treatment for their esophageal cancer before surgery (chemotherapy, immunotherapy, or radiation therapy—sometimes all together), undergo complex esophageal surgery with reconstruction of their anatomy, and then slowly begin eating again. From there, it's a move into survivorship care, which is a combination of chronic symptom management, cancer surveillance, and targeted, focused intervention. In Houston, the support group had helped tremendously with that, creating a de facto survivorship program. The problem is that most places at that time, Mayo included, didn't have a formal survivorship program in place. Instead, after the acute phase of their treatment, patients were often left to deal with medical oncologists, surgeons, and a variety of other providers in a manner that was fragmented at best. Our patients would travel back to their homes and return to their local providers for maintenance care. Patients bounced between specialists and generalists as they tried to find someone with the knowledge and experience to take care of their issues—and, yes, who could understand their new anatomy and digestion.

I once had a gastroenterologist tell one of my esophagectomy patients that his terrible dumping was because I cut his vagal nerve during the cancer surgery. Cutting the vagal nerve, uniformly standard when cancer is the diagnosis, is an essential step in every esophagectomy. All surgeons do it. It is described in all of the textbooks and is the standard of care today. But this gastroenterologist made it sound as if I had done something wrong. The patient was alarmed—understandably so—and he came to me angry, thinking I had made a technical error. This is just one example of how aftercare can be mismanaged, confusing, and difficult.

Patients fare better when they receive appropriate care in a supportive network. When we surgeons and providers stay tethered to the people we treat, we can better understand the impact of our surgical decisions on our patients, as well as get a more realistic view of survival rates. Wanting to stay in touch with my patients in my new job, I cobbled together a combination of resources, including Mayo Clinic Connect (we created a specific esophageal cancer section within that blog and generated content for it on a routine basis); a Mayo Clinic Florida-based, patient-driven virtual support group (meeting regularly on Zoom); and a national Esophageal Cancer Education Foundation patient-driven support group, also virtual. In addition, I established our survivorship care team and a Facebook page for survivors to associate with one another, and participated on as many of these social media platforms as I could.

Since I have insomnia, I would monitor the banter in the middle of the night, adding my two cents where appropriate, correcting egregiously wrong advice. That said, I have to be careful when I'm on social media because I don't want to give specific medical advice to someone who is not my patient. When I jump in online I'm always very careful, so I say things like "You may want to think about X" or "Have you considered Y?" or "You should talk to your doctor about this. She'll have a perspective that will help." Still, I think it's important to be active when I can, because—unfortunately—many people give far too much credence to what is discussed on social media platforms, often relying on them as their go-to source of information.

I've witnessed one patient suggest that another eat ice cream to combat weight loss. (Actually, I've seen this more than once.) This is bad advice on so many levels. Not only are some patients lactose intolerant after surgery, but others might suffer massive dumping from eating sugary ice cream, causing them to be even more malnourished than before. "Eat popcorn" is another popular suggestion as a way to absorb the bile reflux. But the bile reflux could be more than an uncomfortable side effect. It could be a sign that something is very wrong. Furthermore, many patients struggle with ingesting anything that swells in their newly constructed esophagus, which is made from a stapled tube of stomach tissue. Rice, bread, and popcorn might not go down so well and may cause swelling within the tube, which no longer has peristalsis to push the food down into the stomach. While popcorn may absorb some of the bile and make the patient temporarily feel better, it is not really recommended. Anyone having bile go into their airway needs to be evaluated by a team to determine why that is happening, instead of self-soothing with popcorn.

Unfortunately, too many patients don't realize this and instead come up with all kinds of home remedies that they share online in an effort to help. Not being medical experts, they miss the gravity of the situation, sometimes with grave consequences. Patients tend to think that what worked for them will work for everyone. That's definitely not the case. Others may just give worthless or inaccurate information. And then there are the people who use themselves as a reference point for other people's illness. I see this a lot these days when people get COVID and then say it felt like "just a bad cold." That may be true for a great many people, but it's not true for all, and to assume that the experience of an illness is the same for everyone does those who are suffering a great disservice. Sure, most people act with the best of intentions, but friendly advice can be dangerous if it stops a person from going to a doctor who can recognize the problem, diagnose it, and find a solution to make things better.

At the Houston support group I was always there to serve as a backup for my patients. I preferred not to take center stage, so to speak. But I was there to intervene if clarification was needed, and I could make sure our members left the group with sound advice and up-to-date information. The internet, on the other hand, is like the Wild West. And there's usually no sheriff on social media. That's why I'm careful about the resources I give my patients. I stand by Mayo Connect—we're all really proud of it. Its blog is monitored to make sure the information there is correct. But still, I felt my patients needed more.

Especially when it comes to cancer, information without context can be baffling, leaving patients vulnerable and confused. And too much information can be overwhelming and cause people to freeze up. They don't know what to do when they're in trouble; they may even have difficulty recognizing when they *are* in trouble. It may sound strange, the idea that patients may know not if they are actually struggling. But cancer is a new country, and people have to make their way through it as best as they can, learning new customs as they go.

Some believe that dumping or diarrhea will always be a part of life, not realizing that there are things that can be done to improve it. Others might have bile that comes into their mouth because their reconstructed esophagus is twisted, has become what we call redundant, or has herniated. Being able to name their issues, to understand how they are doing compared with how they actually *could* be doing, is vital to a patient's health and quality of life. Having a contextual understanding of their issue may also protect patients from being told to "just tolerate" their symptoms by providers who do not understand the issue at hand.

That is another reason patients with esophageal cancer should be treated by doctors who consider this disease their specialty. Only someone immersed in this world can truly understand the array of symptoms and what might be done about them. Survival is a wonderful goal, one that we all strive to reach. But quantity of life without quality, well . . . that's not how anybody wants to live. Too often people survive surgery but end up with complications or symptoms that severely impact their lives, and they don't know where to turn.

One man I knew had made it through his esophagectomy only to experience the worst reflux imaginable. When he went back to visit his own doctor, he was told that he had undergone a complicated surgery that most people don't survive, so he should consider it a gift that he had not had any major complications. The insensitivity of that statement makes me see red. I wouldn't consider reflux so bad that it's threatening your life to be a gift. When someone who has defied the odds is told that they should be grateful, the burden is real. It can be oppressive and, frankly, damaging to a patient who is being treated like an ungrateful child who needs to eat his vegetables because there are other children starving in the world.

A friend of mine had a beloved niece who was in a terrible car accident. The young mother was only twenty-eight when her car flipped over three times and she had to be airlifted to a hospital. Cassandra spent nine weeks in a coma, and many more weeks after that in intensive care. Barbara, my friend, was distraught. She didn't have any children of her own and was very close to her niece. The weeks and months that Cassandra was in the hospital were nerve-racking, but luckily Barbara had some very good friends who helped her through. They checked in on Barbara to see not just how her niece was doing but also how she was coping in the midst of such prolonged uncertainty and stress. "I don't know how I would have made it without them," Barbara said. "So many people showing up for me made me realize just how fortunate I am. Especially my buddy David. He was a rock."

Cassandra made a remarkable recovery, much to everyone's great relief. But she suffered a traumatic brain injury (TBI) and severe damage to her optic nerve, which left her legally blind. She could no longer drive, and reading gave her headaches. The TBI affected her memory and sometimes her thought processes and her mood. Cassandra's life became much smaller. But when Barbara mentioned this to David one day, he became impatient with her.

"Remember when this first happened? All you kept saying was 'Please don't let her die . . . please don't let her die.' Well, she's alive, now, isn't she? Shouldn't you be grateful?"

Barbara was dumbstruck. Yes, that was what she had said in the early days after the accident. And yes, she'd be the first to admit how grateful she was. But as with so many catastrophic events and illnesses, there was no going back to the way things were. Everyone was doing their best, but the whole family was forced to deal with a new normal that sometimes was difficult. People can be grateful to be on the other side of a large medical event and still struggle. It's not always a life-or-death situation; it's not always black or white. We have to live in the gray area, where we acknowledge that the worst hasn't happened, but we may still have to cope with some pretty devastating consequences—day after day after day.

The burden of gratitude, indeed.

I worried about the long-term survivorship of my new patients at Mayo. Would they struggle alone without a support group, without some way to keep in touch and understand the context of what was happening to them? Struggling in silence can lead to depression—and, even worse, suicide. (The suicide rate in this patient population is abnormally high.) We needed a better way to identify who was in trouble and who was doing well, some way to gather information and put it in a centralized place.

But how to do that?

I thought of virtual healthcare. Popular even before the COVID-19 pandemic, virtual healthcare (including telehealth doctor's visits and digital information exchange) has provided patients with the ability to receive care in their own home. Virtual healthcare is a real boon to the patient, who no longer has to be bound to the physical hospital. In the case of Mayo, to which so many people travel from around the country—indeed, from around the world—it means we can keep an eye on our patients from afar. Was there a way to make use of either virtual or digital resources to aid with survivorship care, a way to help cancer survivors manage the physical and emotional changes they experience after treatment? After all, we set out to cure, connect, and transform.

The medical community is no stranger to big data. Big data has enabled research and clinical trials to identify populations at risk for a variety of health problems. We rely on it to detect patterns and to turn information analysis into actionable knowledge for meaningful change in precision medicine. We also use it to guide future decisions and make policy changes. And every day we're learning more. We now have the ability to understand numbers and patient data to the extent that we are often overwhelmed with information. We have national databases that score outcomes of individuals and institutions against one another, giving a star rating to those that stand out. We have dashboards that can track infections, complications, readmissions, and other hospital factors to improve outcomes. We have conversational AI-enabled technology that can ask patients about their symptoms and then help them look for resources. Surely all of these technologies could extend to survivorship care.

Perhaps. But did our patients really want more technology or another survey?

I had been thinking of developing a questionnaire to give to my patients at Mayo, something that would help me get to know the people I would be treating. I wanted a survey that would help me better understand their needs and where my team could improve. But the catch-22 of it all is that patients are often reluctant to fill them out because of something called "survey fatigue." This is the all-too-real feeling of exasperation, boredom, and indifference we feel due to the overwhelming number of surveys we're asked to complete. At Mayo Clinic, we started getting feedback that patients were complaining about too many surveys. Now we have a committee to review and approve them, in order to prevent patients from being burdened. It's a worthwhile group that also screens the surveys to make sure there's not too much overlap with other surveys the patient might be offered. It may feel a little Kafkaesque, establishing a committee to study surveys that people don't really want to fill out in the first place, but I believe feedback is essential to giving patients what *they* want. We can't make assumptions based on our experience. I talk to my patients, of course. But the benefit of a survey is that it provides aggregate information that gives us a big-picture view of patients' concerns and tells us what they value most. Still, we have to be respectful of what we ask and mindful of the fact that many people have a great mistrust of these institution-generated questionnaires.

Our patients' time is valuable, and if they're going to become engaged with their own healthcare and complete a survey, they're going to want something back. I hear this all the time. I certainly heard it in the support group. Nothing is more frustrating to a patient than to provide information without actually finding out what the purpose of it is, basically completing something that just goes into a black hole. I had been a patient at a wellness clinic for post-menopausal care where I was given an extensive questionnaire on depression and anxiety. At the time I wasn't sleeping and had a reasonable amount of anxiety about it. Nothing ever came from my survey, and no one ever asked me if I was truly anxious and how they could help. This is how trust is eroded. Surveys need to be used, and patients need to see that they're used. I hoped my answers in the surveys would raise a red flag. Instead, they were ignored. I am not even sure my survey went under anyone's eyes.

A good survey that is put to good use is tremendously valuable. Was there a way to put together something that would allow our patients to track their symptoms and progress, one that would let them know if they were getting better or worse after the introduction of a new procedure or protocol? What's more, could it be used as a metric whereby patients could compare themselves with other survivors and tell physicians how they are doing in a standardized way? I thought back to what the business educator Peter Drucker once said: "If you can't measure it, you can't manage it."

That was a lightbulb moment, if ever there was one. And it was with this in mind—measuring and managing the survivorship of our patients—that we developed the Upper Digestive Disease App. Available on iOS and Android, the app is an elegant solution used by patients and healthcare providers alike. The UDD App asks the patients questions, scores and color-codes their problems, then connects our patients to a standardized monitoring system. Patients can even export their report card to their care providers by email. All of this allows tracking of symptoms over time, enabling clinics to access information before a patient even walks in the door. That in turn means that the time we spend with patients can be devoted to solving their problems instead of recognizing or diagnosing them. Saving this time allows providers to serve more people, making more people better.

Clearly, the UDD App grew out of what I learned in the support group. Developed with patient volunteers—we now have around eight hundred people who have participated in the questionnaires in some fashion so far—it is based on what they've told us is important to them during recovery and beyond. We started with a baseline questionnaire on paper. *What is your age? Your gender? What was your diagnosis? Did you have surgery, and if so, when?* All the getting-to-know-you data that a medical provider needs. From there, we asked more specific questions about dumping, reflux, heartburn, regurgitation, weight loss, fatigue, overall decline in physical health, decline in mental health, and a myriad of other symptoms pertinent to the care of people with that disease group, or pertinent to the group of symptoms that have been volunteered by patients as the things they care about the most. We have now launched a decentralized clinical trial to offer the UDD App to all patients around the world free of cost while we collect their data for comparative outcomes analysis. We want to improve outcomes for this patient population and know which treatments are better.

On that initial paper-based questionnaire, patients provided us with scores based on their own measurements of the frequency, interference with daily life, and severity of their symptoms. In time, that paper version of the questionnaire became the app. Once we picked the symptoms we wanted to measure, we asked questions in different ways to help measure each symptom domain. This was to make sure we didn't ask questions in a manner that would confuse patients or prompt them to provide an answer they *thought* we were looking for. The first round of inquiry focused on the frequency and severity of symptoms, all in service of three big questions:

- How often do you experience this?
- How severe is it?
- How much does this interfere with your life?

All other questions were contextual. For example, we might ask if a patient had problems swallowing warm or cold liquids, if their symptoms changed when they elevated the head of their bed, or what happened if they ate right before going to sleep. These contextual items help the provider understand what behaviors may influence a patient's symptoms.

From there, we measured the data to understand patterns of answers, making sure we were only measuring one domain at a time. Essentially, we looked at both the scores and the "purity" of each question to figure out how to extract data and put it on a 0-100 scale. Next, we color-coded the scores to give each patient a severity color. We wanted a model everyone was familiar with, so we went with the traffic light theme. Green represents patients who are doing well. Yellow represents those who might need targeted education. Red represents patients who have severe symptoms and who might be in trouble.

At this stage, experts from all disciplines and levels of care provided input, our goal being to help the patient communicate directly with follow-up providers who may not have the same level of experience or expertise in dealing with their cancer. Our experts looked at the questions, the scores, and the domains to determine how they thought patients should be characterized if they were managing them at a clinic. The color-coded scores let patients, their caregivers, and their providers know when they are doing okay and when they need additional in-person support. Patients who score green know they are doing well. Those who score yellow are alerted to the fact that they may need some help to do better—they may, for example, need to be reevaluated, with steps taken to ensure that they begin moving back to green. Those who score in the red zone know that they need a provider review, evaluation, or intervention with a provider visit.

Patients who do not return to Mayo Clinic, or who were never at Mayo to begin with, can take their results back to their local providers to be managed in their local care circles. While the survivorship clinic is specifically for Mayo patients, the UDD App can be utilized by patients all over the world. We wanted to build an app that will help people who have issues with their upper digestive system advocate for themselves with their own physicians and better understand what is happening to them. And that's what we've done. With the app, providers who did not know how to determine whether or not their patients were in trouble will now have an easier time triaging, managing, and tracking progress. Simply put, we have simplified the entire process of triage for these patients and their providers.

Patients who remain within the Mayo system will get the care they need to manage red-zone symptoms. They will be evaluated, undergo diagnostic tests, and be referred to specialists. This intervention is carefully monitored by the survivorship care team with the aim of getting the patient back in the green zone. We stay linked to survivors over time, and each year we connect with them by video visit. I really like doing video visits with my patients because usually the whole family is there. Whether they're scrunched in the same room and on the same screen, or connected around the country on Zoom with each person in their own box on the screen, it's really helpful for me to see my patients' support systems in place. I can answer everyone's questions (I love it when those questions are well coordinated), doing what I can to ensure that my patients have the necessary medical support to continue in their survivorship. Legally, according to the Centers for Medicare and Medicaid Services, when a patient becomes disconnected from their provider for three years, the patient-provider relationship is considered disintegrated, and they can no longer connect by video for follow-up visits. Our virtual, digitally enabled clinic, which uses the app as a triage tool, solves that problem as well.

Necessity really is the mother of invention. The greater our needs are, the greater the solution needs to be. Certainly, the more creative we have to be. We have begun to solve those problems one by one. Now we are in the process of connecting the dots for our patients, encouraging them to utilize the app and engage with their providers as their own advocates.

Survivorship is ongoing. As my former patient Rayna Huber posted on social media in June for Cancer Survivor Month: "A cancer diagnosis and traumatic treatment has long-term effects. From the life-long changes to the body, from the PTSD from seeing so many doctors, there is a reason cancer patients are referred to as warriors. It's like coming back from battle, only your adversary is your body."

Seventeen

Tools of the Trade

make it a point never to leave the room until all of my patients' questions are answered, which means that sometimes I run late in clinic. I've also been known to overbook my calendar to accommodate patients who need to be seen, which can make clinic time last longer. This can make things difficult for the staff, but they understand how important it is for patients to have a sense of confidence and comfort. I never want to be the kind of doctor who stands at the door with their hand on the knob trying to leave as a patient begs to have just one more question answered. I hate the thought of someone waiting weeks to get answers. I've been there myself. It's not pleasant.

But I'll admit, it can cause problems.

I was running late one day and had kept a patient waiting. More than one, as it happens. The few remaining patients had started talking to one another in the waiting room. Likely it began with polite smiles, sympathetic glances, and a few benign comments about the weather. From there it would go a little deeper, one person testing the waters with another to see how much the other wanted to open up. This must have been a chummy group, because they shared information about jobs and family, about who did what for a living and who lived where. I find in the clinic that when the conversation turns to geography, it's not long before a group—no matter how large or small—determines who has traveled the farthest. Turns out that it was my last patient who garnered the award that day. It was one he'd rather not have had, however, because he was scheduled to fly home that night. And his doctor—me—was behind schedule.

Asaad had undergone an esophagectomy several years before. He kept going back to the surgeon who performed the operation to tell him how bad the reflux was. Asaad would wake up in the middle of the night drowning in liquids that came from his stomach (part of which had been surgically moved into his chest) and would aspirate the contents back into his lungs. This caused him to get sick and miss work. Asaad had missed so much work, in fact, that he was afraid he was about to lose his job. If he lost his job, he would lose his health insurance. Then he'd really be in trouble. Although he was in financial peril, he scraped money together to buy a ticket to fly to Mayo Clinic to see me. He had heard I liked to solve complex esophageal problems, and he knew he needed help. This was a desperate last attempt to try to find a solution.

Asaad was in a time crunch the day he came to see me, so when he saw that I was running late he got on the phone to find out if he had any other flight options. While this was happening, the patient scheduled before him offered to give Asaad his slot. We all wanted the same thing: for Asaad to have his consultation with me and to make his flight home. Some creative problem-solving was necessary, that's for sure.

Well, it turned out that the only way to make this happen was for me to drive Asaad to the airport and talk to him on the way. It would be a driving consultation, of sorts, where instead of sitting behind a clipboard I'd be sitting behind a wheel. Asaad had been stressed in the clinic waiting room, but once he clicked the seatbelt in my car, he let his guard down. He told me how he had been feeling suicidal from all of the pain he was in, the aspiration events, and the fact that he was so close to losing his job. He didn't feel heard by his surgeon. It seemed to him that no one really cared about how much he was suffering. The surgeon at one point told him, "You're really lucky to have survived such a deadly surgery. Just be glad you're alive." With no other friends or acquaintances who had undergone the same surgery or had a similar frame of reference, Asaad believed the surgeon for a while. Maybe this was as good as it gets, he thought.

Asaad's symptoms were nearly impossible to tolerate, and he worried that one day he would aspirate so badly he would end up on a ventilator. The fear and frustration in his eyes were more than I could stand. I thought long and hard about what to do. Asaad's pyloric valve had been cut and the position of his stomach in the chest was causing the reflux. It wasn't just acid reflux—it was bile reflux. I knew this because I had been able to review his case before he came to the clinic.

Asaad had answered the survey that was the outgrowth of the support group. The UDD app enabled me to use his answers to help determine which problem was causing him the most distress. That the assessment was done even before he came to the clinic made it easier for me to spend my time and attention talking to him in an effort to solve the problem, rather than just figuring out what the problem was. Unfortunately, when doctors see patients in the clinic without having been able to review answers to questions like those on the app, they might have to spend about thirty to forty-five minutes before they even get close to the real issue. Because of the thirty minutes Asaad took to answer the eighty questions *before* we met, we were already ahead of the game.

It was no surprise he was in trouble. His dysphagia, pain, dumping, and reflux scores were some of the most terrible we had measured. Comparing Asaad's scores with other patients' scores—as well as with those that benchmarked where experts at Mayo thought they should be—I knew that the other surgeon was wrong in his assessment. Asaad shouldn't have to just "bear it" and deal with the symptoms. Those symptoms weren't compatible with a good life; they were life-threatening. They weren't even normal for a patient who had undergone an esophagectomy. My patient deserved better. But what to do? I racked my brain for days trying to find a solution.

Then it came to me.

Rerouting the bowel would stop Asaad's reflux. And I could help the stomach to empty by attaching the jejunum to the bottom of the stomach, which would help drain the stomach conduit. (That was what one of my old surgical mentors, Dr. J. P. Wilson, from Georgia Baptist Hospital, referred to as the "living sucker" surgery.) All of my general surgery training had come in handy. I had been taught not just what surgeries to do in what circumstances but to think for myself and solve problems that weren't in the textbook. And the app helped.

Quantifying his misery with a tool, my new patient provided us with valuable information. That information helped us determine what symptom we needed to tackle first. The severity of Asaad's reflux and aspiration prompted me to get a swallow test to see where things were hanging up. From there, I was able to build a plan. I suggested my "living sucker" surgery to him, but I made sure to tell him that it might make his dumping problem worse. He chose to proceed. I reassured him that if the dumping worsened after we got the reflux under control, we would then work on addressing that issue. We were able to methodically solve each problem and help him reclaim his life.

Asaad had spent years wondering why he felt so terrible and why no one really seemed to understand how bad off he was. I was so grateful that he sought a second opinion. Piece by piece, we put him back together again and made him whole. He's back at work now, not worrying about losing his job; getting on with his life. Things aren't perfect, but his scores are much better (much more green than yellow or red), and when I see him now, he often smiles and always looks good. Sometimes he even jokingly asks for a ride back to the airport.

When I think back on this case, I realize that a big part of the problem was that Asaad didn't know he was an outlier. He didn't know how to compare his symptom profile against those of others who had undergone similar surgeries. Neither did his surgeon. I thought about sending the scores to this other doctor, and then I realized perhaps everyone should have access to this. As I mentioned earlier, we've now made the app available to everyone for free, worldwide. Even if their doctors may not know how to solve their problem, at least they can know what the problem is and how to begin to solve it. This was a gift built upon listening to the voices of my patients for years while conducting the support group meetings. Teaching my patients to advocate for themselves, giving them a voice, and allowing them to present something in an objective way that is measured consistently seems like a pretty good gift.

Eighteen

Full Circle

There is power in the stories we tell. When we share our narratives, we reach outside our own experience and make ourselves vulnerable. We learn from and take strength from one another. This is one of the basic principles of support. Whether you are in a group setting or one-on-one, sharing your situation with others can help you process, grieve, and begin to find solutions. Only when we let people see who we are and what we're going through can we build a connection. Stories open us up to what's unique in everyone, the nuanced shades of gray instead of the indelible lines of black and white.

I am grateful to have been able to play a small part in the lives of a great many people. It has been a privilege and a gift, one that has provided me with tremendous insight into my own life. It's not just because dealing with cancer patients, many of whom don't have a lot of time left, encourages a perspective I might never otherwise have gained. And it's not just that my patients have taught me meaning, that they've shown me how to appreciate even the most mundane moments—they have. It's more than that. It's that being forced to deal with illness, being up against the hard truth that everyone's time is limited, makes you realize pretty quickly what's important and what's not. My patients have provided me with a compass in life. Connecting to them has made me understand the struggles everyone faces and how we're all so much better when we deal with them together.

At this point in my career, I can say unequivocally that the more connected I am to my patients, the better I can serve and support them. I will do anything I can to make my patients' lives better, but that will be possible only if I listen to what it is they really want. And here's the irony: what is true for our patients is also true for those of us who tend to them. Now that I'm two-thirds of the way through my career and have had a chance to connect the dots, it's become clear to me that the best practices for our patients are also the best practices for providers. What we all need is connection and support, the ability to speak with honesty and respect and without fear of repercussions. But we need to have a system that makes room for that.

I think the thing that's most broken in our society at large, not just in our medical institutions, is that so many of us are acting from a place of self-preservation. So many divisive forces are tugging people every which way that they feel the only thing to do is to protect themselves. I see this in young physicians and surgeons who are trying to give themselves a better quality of life. That is, of course, completely understandable. And it's a laudable goal, considering the tremendous stress they are under. But a side effect of this is that by protecting their own time, more and more providers are switching off and disconnecting from patients. Our frenzied healthcare system makes this possible, if not desirable.

With practices getting larger and administrators growing in number and power, and with so many of them operating under the auspices of behemoth corporations, providers find it easier to detach and retreat. I'm not saying that we should always be tethered to our hospitals or our patients. I came up under that system and I know how burdensome it was. But we were allied with our patients in a way that has largely disappeared these days. We got to know them, *really* got to know them. And we understood their suffering because we understood them. It's empathy born out of experience, and it has spurred in many of us a deep desire to alleviate the pain and suffering of those in our care.

The system has to support this connection. And it must support patients and providers alike. I have seen leaders draw a target on the backs of physicians. I have seen those same doctors lose confidence and conviction as their careers and their lives have unraveled. We have got to figure out a better way to sustain healthcare and healthcare providers, because the current model is not working. There's no room for empathy when profit is the main motive, when the goal of an institution is to get bigger rather than better. We need to appreciate the contribution diverse teams bring to the table. We must pause for a minute to listen and understand one another. It is in this understanding that we grow and learn from one another's experience.

But all is not lost.

Every day I see young healthcare providers who want to make a difference, who are trying to navigate the current system in a way that benefits their patients and themselves. They know that there is tremendous power in their everyday actions—that, as the saying goes, you can't save the world, but you can make a big difference in the world of the person in front of you. So many people in healthcare live by those words. If only we all did.

I feel as if I've come full circle since the days at Houston Methodist, when I started the support group. I built the group because I felt I didn't have enough time with my patients, I needed to figure out how to be more economical with my time, to find solutions to what seemed an insurmountable problem. The support group became a lifeline, one that fueled my passion for helping patients and gave me an incredibly strong sense of purpose and direction. It gave me so much. And now I want to return the favor. There is power in the stories of my patients and colleagues. Within those stories lies the answer.

Acknowledgments

would like to acknowledge the incredible support I received from Brenda Copeland to organize my thoughts and tell my story in a way that conveys my passion for my patients. And to Daniela Rapp and the team at Mayo Press, thank you so much for the opportunity to share this with the world.

My professors and colleagues from The Hockaday School, The University of Texas, Emory University, Morehouse School of Medicine, Georgia Baptist, Baylor College of Medicine, MD Anderson Cancer Center, Houston Methodist Hospital (especially Elaine Jordan, Min Kim, and Andrea McNeil), and Mayo Clinic have taught me so much throughout my career. I am forever grateful for the Mayo Clinic Center for Digital Health teams I have had the privilege and honor of working with, specifically Radhika Alla, Brad Leibovich, Pranav Joshipura, Publicis Sapient and Mark Schumacher. The UDD App lab team members, especially Karly Pierson, Kathleen Yost, Minji Lee, and Mohamad Khair Abou Chaar, have taught me about patient-centered research. I am grateful for my surrogate families of ASA, ISDE, ESTS, STS, STSA, WTS, and AATS. To the Nassef 10 Tower Nurses, support staff, and especially my OR crew, Janet, Jaymie, Keri, and Cassie et al.—you taught me what it is to have a highly functioning and effective team. For my residents, thank you for all you have taught me and for going out into the world to change it for the better. A special thanks to Mark Allen, Summer Allen, Mara Antonoff, Leah

Backhus, Atta Behfar, Tom Bower, Lisa Brown, Nav Buttar, Charles Clayton, Yolonda Colson, Joe Coselli, Juan Crestanello, Tommy D'Amico, Elizabeth David, Joe Dearani, Emily DeGrazia, Randy DeMartino, Karen Dickinson, Donna and Eric Dozois, Brooks Edwards, Melanie Edwards, Camille Evans, Bridget Fahy, Shamiram Feinglass, Stephanie Fuller, Travis Grotz, Lance Haley, Sally Hudspeth, Chris Lucius, Mike Maddaus, Linda Martin, Doug Mathisen, Natalie Mauldin, Leo Misenbach, Kendall and Preston Moister, Daniela Molena, Victor Montori, Laura Moore, Frank Nichols, John Noseworthy, Peter Noseworthy, Jamie and Pam Packer, Tom Pagenkopf, Rene Petersen, Alberto Pochettino, Dan and Katharine Price, Mike Reardon, Jenna Romano, Katie Ruddy, Sahar Saddoughi, Netu Sarkaria, Vicky and Rafa Sierra, Chase Sims, Elizabeth Stephens, Claudia Tabini, Luis Tapias, Vinod Thourani, S. Rob Todd, Mark Truty, Ara Vaporciyan, Tom Varghese, Mac and Cynthia Walker, Bernie and Kathryn Weber, Doug Wood, Kazu Yasufuku, and so many more of you who daily inspire me. For our core local family and Rochester friend group who helped keep us sane and have fun in the frozen tundra. And, of course, my large, complex, and often confusing but incredibly supportive family—especially my husband, Matt Blackmon, and our precious kids, Grace, Jake, and Sam. My Mom (Leigh Jones Garrett), of course. And my brother Lance Haley and all the Haleys, Watsons, Blackmons, Garretts, Bagwells, Rachofskys, and the family-by-choice extras.

There are so many people I cannot name but you know who you are. No one does this kind of work without a village of support.

Resources

A great many books and resources have influenced my life and career and the writing of this book. I am pleased to share a selection of them with my readers in the hope that they may prove as helpful to you as they have been to me.

Of General Interest

Collins, Jim. *Great by Choice: Uncertainty, Chaos, and Luck—Why Some Thrive Despite Them All* (Harper Business, 2011).

Csikszentmihalyi, Mihaly. *Flow: The Psychology of Optimal Experience* (Harper & Row, 1990).

Duckworth, Angela. *Grit: The Power of Passion and Perseverance* (Scribner, 2016).

Gawande, Atul. *Being Mortal: Medicine and What Matters in the End* (Metropolitan Books, 2014).

Grenny, Joseph, Kerry Patterson, Ron McMillan, Al Switzler, and Emily Gregory. *Crucial Conversations: Tools for Talking When Stakes Are High* (McGraw Hill, 2022).

Montori, Victor. *Why We Revolt: A Patient Revolution for Careful and Kind Care* (Patient Revolution, 2017).

Porath, Christine. *Mastering Community: The Surprising Ways Coming Together Moves Us from Surviving to Thriving* (Grand Central Publishing, 2023).

Werner, D. Judith K. *ReMarkable: The Grit and Grace of Mark Clifton* (Amazon Publishing, 2017).

Of Interest to Healthcare Providers

Drebing, C. *Leading Peer Support and Self-Help Groups: A Pocket Resource for Peer Specialists and Support Group Facilitators* (Lulu.com, 2016).

Edmondson, A. C., & Bransby, D. P. Psychological Safety Comes of Age: Observed Themes in an Established Literature. *Annual Review of Organizational Psychology and Organizational Behavior 10*(1): 55-78.

Edmondson, A. C., & Harvey, J.. *Extreme Teaming: Lessons in Complex, Cross-Sector Leadership* (Emerald Group Publishing, 2017).

Krueger, R. A. *Focus Groups: A Practical Guide for Applied Research* (SAGE Publications, 1988).

Kurtz, L. F. *Self-Help and Support Groups: A Handbook for Practitioners* (SAGE Publications, 1997).

Miller, J. E. *Effective Support Groups: How to Plan, Design, Facilitate, and Enjoy Them* (Willowgreen Publishing, 1998).

Schopler, J. H., & Galinsky, M. J. *Support Groups: Current Perspectives on Theory and Practice* (Taylor & Francis, 2014).

Resources for Patients

American Joint Committee on Cancer (AJCC): https://www.facs.org/quality-programs

CanCare: https://www.cancare.org

Esophageal Cancer Action Network: https://ecan.org

Esophageal Cancer Education Foundation (ECEF): www.fightec.org

Mayo Clinic Esophageal Cancer Support Group: EsophagealSurvivors@mayo.edu

National Comprehensive Cancer Network (NCCN): https://www.nccn.org/patientresources/patient-resources

Resources for Healthcare Providers

Antonoff, M. B., Stephens, E. H., & Blackmon, S. H. (2020). Meeting the Educational Needs of an Increasingly Diverse Surgical Workforce. *JAMA Surgery, 155*(6), 533-534. https://doi.org/10.1001/jamasurg.2020.0097

Brunelli, A., Blackmon, S. H., Sentürk, M., Cavalheri, V., & Pompili, C. (2022). Patient-centred care in thoracic surgery: a holistic approach—A review of the subjects of enhanced recovery after surgery, rehabilitation, pain management and patient-reported outcome measures in thoracic surgery. *Journal of Thoracic Disease, 14*(2), 546-552. https://doi.org/10.21037/jtd-21-1763

Ceppa, D. P., Antonoff, M. B., Tong, B. C., Timsina, L., Ikonomidis, J. S., Worrell, S. G., Stephens, E. H., Gillaspie, E. A., Schumacher, L., Molena, D., Kane,

L. C., Blackmon, S., & Donington, J. S. (2022). 2020 Women in Thoracic Surgery Update on the Status of Women in Cardiothoracic Surgery. *The Annals of Thoracic Surgery, 113*(3), 918–925. https://doi.org/10.1016/j.athorac sur.2021.03.091

Ceppa, D. P., Dolejs, S. C., Boden, N., Phelan, S., Yost, K. J., Donington, J., Naunheim, K. S., & Blackmon, S. (2020). Sexual Harassment and Cardiothoracic Surgery: #UsToo?. *The Annals of Thoracic Surgery, 109*(4), 1283–1288. https://doi.org/10.1016/j.athoracsur.2019.07.009

Chaar, M. K. A., Yost, K. J., Lee, M. K., Chlan, L. L., Ghosh, K., Hudspeth, L. A., Jatoi, A., Ruddy, K. J., Santore, L. A., & Blackmon, S. H. (2023). Developing & Integrating a Mobile Application Tool into a Survivorship Clinic for Esophageal Cancer Patients. *Journal of Thoracic Disease, 15*(4), 2240–2252. https://doi.org/10.21037/jtd-22-1343

D'Souza, R. S., Sims, C. R., 3rd, Andrijasevic, N., Stewart, T. M., Curry, T. B., Hannon, J. A., Blackmon, S., Cassivi, S. D., Shen, R. K., Reisenauer, J., Wigle, D., & Brown, M. J. (2021). Pulmonary Complications in Esophagectomy Based on Intraoperative Fluid Rate: A Single-Center Study. *Journal of Cardiothoracic and Vascular Anesthesia, 35*(10), 2952–2960. https://doi.org /10.1053/j.jvca.2021.01.006

Elkbuli, A., Sutherland, M., Shepherd, A., Kinslow, K., Liu, H., Ang, D., & McKenney, M. (2022). Factors Influencing US Physician and Surgeon Suicide Rates 2003 to 2017: Analysis of the CDC-National Violent Death Reporting System. *Annals of Surgery, 276*(5), e370–e376. https://doi.org /10.1097/SLA.0000000000004575

Faruqi, F., Ruddy, K. J., & Blackmon, S. (2021). Integrative Approaches to Minimize Peri-operative Symptoms. *Current Oncology Reports, 23*(6), 73. https://doi.org/10.1007/s11912-021-01051-9

Hasan, I. S., Mahajan, N., Viehman, J., Allen, M. S., Cassivi, S. D., Lee, M. K., Nichols, F. C., Pierson, K., Reisenauer, J. S., Shen, R. K., Wigle, D. A., & Blackmon, S. H. (2020). Predictors of Patient-Reported Reflux After Esophagectomy. *The Annals of Thoracic Surgery, 110*(4), 1160–1166. https:// doi.org/10.1016/j.athoracsur.2020.03.127

Kane, L., Litle, V. R., Blackmon, S. H., & Yanagawa, J. (2021). The National and Global Impact of "Women in Thoracic Surgery." *Journal of Thoracic Disease, 13*(1), 432–438. https://doi.org/10.21037/jtd-20-2225

Maddaus M. (2023). Cardiothoracic Surgeons as Second Victims: We, Too, Are at Risk. *The Journal of Thoracic and Cardiovascular Surgery, 166*(3), 881–889. https://doi.org/10.1016/j.jtcvs.2022.11.010

National Comprehensive Cancer Network (NCCN): https://www.nccn.org/guidelines/nccn-guidelines

Olive, J. K., Iranpour, N., Luc, J. G. Y., Preventza, O. A., Blackmon, S. H., & Antonoff, M. B. (2020). Representation of Women in the Southern Thoracic Surgical Association: Evidence for Positive Change. *The Annals of Thoracic Surgery, 110*(5), 1739–1744. https://doi.org/10.1016/j.athoracsur.2020.02.023

Olive, J. K., Preventza, O. A., Blackmon, S. H., & Antonoff, M. B. (2020). Representation of Women in The Society of Thoracic Surgeons Authorship and Leadership Positions. *The Annals of Thoracic Surgery, 109*(5), 1598–1604. https://doi.org/10.1016/j.athoracsur.2019.07.069

Shemanski, K. A., Ding, L., Kim, A. W., Blackmon, S. H., Wightman, S. C., Atay, S. M., Starnes, V. A., & David, E. A. (2021). Gender Representation Among Leadership at National and Regional Cardiothoracic Surgery Organizational Annual Meetings. *The Journal of Thoracic and Cardiovascular Surgery, 161*(3), 733–744. https://doi.org/10.1016/j.jtcvs.2020.11.157

Trudell, A. M., Frankel, W. C., Luc, J. G. Y., Blackmon, S. H., Kane, L., Varghese, T. K., Jr, & Antonoff, M. B. (2022). Enhancing Support for Women in Cardiothoracic Surgery Through Allyship and Targeted Initiatives. *The Annals of Thoracic Surgery, 113*(5), 1676–1683. https://doi.org/10.1016/j.athoracsur.2021.06.064

Wible P. (2018, January 18). What I've Learned from My Tally of 757 Doctor Suicides. *The Washington Post.* https://www.washingtonpost.com/national/health-science/what-ive-learned-from-my-tally-of-757-doctor-suicides/2018/01/12/b0ea9126-eb50-11e7-9f92-10a2203f6c8d_story.html

Notes

Introduction

1. Thoracic surgery is any kind of surgery that occurs on or inside the chest. Cardiothoracic surgery includes heart and aortic surgery, and is sometimes referred to as thoracic surgery. To delineate the difference between cardiac surgery and thoracic surgery, some surgeons use the term general thoracic surgery. This terminology has confused surgeons and patients for decades.

One

1. Vinnakota, A., Idrees, J. J., Rosinski, B. F., Tucker, N. J., Roselli, E. E., Pettersson, G. B., Vekstein, A. M., Stewart, R. D., Raja, S., & Svensson, L. G. (2019). Outcomes of Repair of Kommerell Diverticulum. *The Annals of Thoracic Surgery, 108*(6), 1745–1750. https://doi.org/10.1016/j.athoracsur.2019.04.122.
2. Verstegen, M. H. P., Bouwense, S. A. W., van Workum, F., Ten Broek, R., Siersema, P. D., Rovers, M., & Rosman, C. (2019). Management of Intrathoracic and Cervical Anastomotic Leakage After Esophagectomy for Esophageal Cancer: A Systematic Review. *World Journal of Emergency Surgery : WJES, 14,* 17. https://doi.org/10.1186/s13017-019-0235-4.

Two

1. Edmondson, A. C., Bohmer, R. M. J., & Pisano, G. P. (2001, October). Speeding Up Team Learning. *Harvard Business Review.* https://hbr.org/2001/10/speeding-up-team-learning.

Three

1. Maddaus M. (2023). Cardiothoracic Surgeons as Second Victims: We, Too, Are at Risk. *The Journal of Thoracic and Cardiovascular Surgery, 166*(3), 881–889. https://doi.org/10.1016/j.jtcvs.2022.11.010.

Five

1. American Cancer Society. (2023, January 12). *Key Statistics for Breast Cancer*. https://www.cancer.org/cancer/breast-cancer/about/how-common-is-breast-cancer.html.
2. American Cancer Society. (2023, January 12). *Key Statistics for Soft Tissue Sarcomas*. https://www.cancer.org/cancer/types/soft-tissue-sarcoma/about/key-statistics.html.

Six

1. Centers for Disease Control and Prevention. (2019, August 7). Caregiving for Family and Friends—a Public Health Issue. https://www.cdc.gov/aging/caregiving/caregiver-brief.html.
2. National Institute on Aging. (n.d.). *National Health and Aging Trends Study NHATS*. https://www.nia.nih.gov/research/resource/national-health-and-aging-trends-study-nhats.
3. Riffin, C., Van Ness, P. H., Wolff, J. L., & Fried, T. (2019). Multifactorial Examination of Caregiver Burden in a National Sample of Family and Unpaid Caregivers. *Journal of the American Geriatrics Society, 67*(2), 277–283. https://doi.org/10.1111/jgs.15664.

Nine

1. Csikszentmihalyi, M. (2009). *Flow: The Psychology of Optimal Experience*. Harper & Row.
2. Pham, D. T., Stephens, E. H., Antonoff, M. B., Colson, Y. L., Dildy, G. A., Gaur, P., Correa, A. M., Litle, V. R., & Blackmon, S. H. (2014). Birth Trends and Factors Affecting Childbearing Among Thoracic Surgeons. *The Annals of Thoracic Surgery, 98*(3), 890–895. https://doi.org/10.1016/j.athoracsur.2014.05.041.

Ten

1. Mayo Clinic Connect. https://connect.mayoclinic.org/.

Twelve

1. Edmondson, A. C., Harvey, J., & Chesbrough, H. W. (2017). *Extreme Teaming: Lessons in Complex, Cross-Sector Leadership*. Emerald Publishing.
2. Grenny, J., Patterson, K., McMillan, R., Switzler, A., & Gregory, E. (2022). *Crucial Conversations: Tools for Talking When Stakes Are High* (3rd ed.). McGraw Hill.

Thirteen

1. Burkeman, O. (2023). *Four Thousand Weeks: Time Management for Mortals.* Picador.
2. Collins, J. (2010). *Always a Wedding: Beginning, Renewing and Rescuing Marriage.* Xulon Press.
3. Bennetts, L. (1979, May 7). Doctors' Wives: Many Report Marriage Is a Disappointment. *The New York Times.*
4. Pinnacle Health Group. (2000). Physician Statistics Summary (1970–1999). https://www.phg.com/2000/01/physician-statistics-summary.
5. Boyle, Patrick. (2021). Nation's Physician Workforce Evolves: More Women, a Bit Older, and Toward Different Specialties. *AAMC.* https://www.aamc.org/news-insights/nation-s-physician-workforce-evolves-more-women-bit-older-and-toward-different-specialties.

Fourteen

1. Sier, V. Q., Schmitz, R. F., Schepers, A., & van der Vorst, J. R. (2023). Exploring the Surgical Personality. *The Surgeon: Journal of the Royal Colleges of Surgeons of Edinburgh and Ireland, 21*(1), 1–7. https://doi.org/10.1016/j.surge.2022.01.008.
2. Grinspoon, P. (2016, June 5). Up to 15% of Doctors Are Drug Addicts. I Was One of Them. *Los Angeles Times,* https://www.latimes.com/opinion/op-ed/la-oe-grinspoon-addicted-doctors-20160605-snap-story.html.